OTHER ACMI PRESS SELECTIONS

By Colette Aboulker-Muscat

Alone with the One

Mea Culpa: Tales of Resurrection

By Gerald Epstein, M.D.

Healing into Immortality:
A New Spiritual Medicine of Healing Stories and Imagery

Kabbalah for Inner Peace:
Imagery and Insight to Guide You through Your Day

Climbing Jacob's Ladder:
Finding Spiritual Freedom through the Stories of the Bible

Waking Dream Therapy:
Unlocking the Secrets of Self through Dreams and Imagination

Studies in Non-Deterministic Psychology

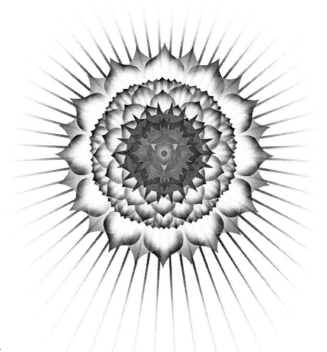

THE
ENCYCLOPEDIA
OF MENTAL IMAGERY

COLETTE ABOULKER-MUSCAT'S 2,100 VISUALIZATION
EXERCISES FOR PERSONAL DEVELOPMENT, HEALING,
AND SELF-KNOWLEDGE

Gerald Epstein, M.D., Editor
Barbarah L. Fedoroff, Editor

THE
ENCYCLOPEDIA
OF MENTAL IMAGERY

Book Cover Design and Interior Layout:
Finn Winterson
wintersondesign.com

This book is not intended as a substitute for medical advice
of physicians. The reader can consult a physician in matters
relating to his or her health and particularly in respect to
any symptoms that may require diagnosis or medical attention.

Library of Congress Cataloging-In-Publication Data
Encyclopedia of mental imagery: Colette Aboulker-Muscat's 2,100
visualization exercises for personal development, healing, and self-knowledge
Gerald Epstein, editor, Barbarah L. Fedoroff, editor. — 1st ed. p. cm.
ISBN-13: 978-1-883148-10-2
Library of Congress Control Number: 2011939982
1. Imagery (Psychology) — Encyclopedias.
I. Aboulker-Muscat, Colette, 1909-2003. II. Epstein, Gerald, 1935-
III. Fedoroff, Barbarah L.
BF367.E54 2012 153.3'2 QBI11-600195

Printed in USA
First edition, 2012
ACMI Press
351 East 84th Street, Suite 10D
New York, New York 10028
Tel: (212) 369-4080
www.acmipress.org

In memory of my beloved teacher Colette
who said to me

"That which is remembered lives on."

As you imagine into your
future ... don't be
satisfied with stories of
how things have gone for others ...
unfold your own myth.

Rumi 13th Century

ACKNOWLEDGEMENTS

This great work has been made possible by a steadfast group of dedicated students of mine who helped gestate and bring this unique project to birth. Their efforts will never be forgotten. Foremost, I am grateful to Ken Guilmartin who inspired me to fulfill this vision by graciously underwriting the costs for this project. My heartfelt thanks to Barbarah and Serge Fedoroff, as well, who transcribed and collated over 2,100 imagery exercises from 1994-2002 while attending my group imagery classes. Thankfully, Serge knew how to use a computer. Barbarah's great editorial energy has been a vital spark in getting this book to see the light of day.

Chaya Deyo assisted Barbarah in her editorial duties. Chaya's clear-headedness and clarity of understanding helped shape the unfolding of this book. I owe much to her insights. Andrea Diamond, my cherished assistant, helped sort out some difficult editorial issues, especially the glossary and editors' introductions. She also assisted with the organization and typing of the final manuscript. A special thanks goes to Harris Dienstfrey, my longtime editor, for reviewing the manuscript. I want to express my thanks to Ms. Tirza Moussaieff, of Jerusalem, who so kindly shared her years of imagery exercises accrued from Colette's imagery classes that I did not have the opportunity to attend. She is surely owed a debt of gratitude. Finally, thanks to my wife, Rachel, whose final editorial inputs and oversight of the production of the book brought this book to light.

Gerald Epstein, M. D.
Founder & Director
American Institute for Mental Imagery

TABLE OF CONTENTS

TABLE OF CONTENTS

TABLE OF CONTENTS

TABLE OF CONTENTS

TABLE OF CONTENTS

TABLE OF CONTENTS

TABLE OF CONTENTS

TABLE OF CONTENTS

TABLE OF CONTENTS

TABLE OF CONTENTS

EDITOR'S INTRODUCTION
GERALD EPSTEIN, M.D.

The Encyclopedia of Mental Imagery: Colette Aboulker-Muscat's 2,100 Visualization Exercises for Personal Development, Healing, and Self-Knowledge is a deep journey into oneself through mental imagery as well as a practice for healing and spiritual growth created by my teacher, of blessed memory, Mme. Colette Aboulker-Muscat. Through imagery, we encourage conversations between our minds and hearts that speak to us in images. These images build a "ladder and scale for your own human development and a platform from which to jump toward the direction of Spirit," noted Colette in her book of poetry.

Colette's work was brought to my attention in 1974 by a young man named Serge, who I met at a Japanese zendo in Jerusalem, where we were sitting in Zen meditation. He was cured of depression by a method he termed mental imagery of which I had no knowledge. His encouragement led me to meet Colette to learn more about this potentially remarkable treatment method.

Within five minutes of conversing with her, I had an epiphany that changed the course of my life. As we exchanged a few remarks about mental imagery, I recounted that Freud's explanation to analysts about using his technique of "free association" was, in essence, an imagery exercise. In Freud's exercise, the analyst tells the patient to imagine the two of them riding on a train, the patient looking out the window describes to the analyst everything he or she sees. Colette responded by asking, "In what direction does the train go?" I was caught short by this seeming non sequitur. I cautiously said that trains go in a horizontal direction, and I made a horizontal gesture with my hand. Colette made an upward movement with her hand and forearm, saying, "Well, what if the direction were changed to this axis?"

At that moment, I can only describe that I dissolved and became a being of light. The vertical movement seemed to lift me from the horizontal hold of the given, the ordinary patterns of everyday cause and effect. I leapt into freedom and saw that the task of being human was to help realize the freedom to go beyond the given, to the newness that we all are capable of, and to our capacity to renew and re-create. Imagery makes this possible.

Immediately, I became a student of imagination and later an apprentice in mental imagery under Colette's tutelage until 1983. As my understanding of imagination deepened, I joined other students who traveled from around the world for Colette's Group Imagery practice. Here, Colette presented imagery exercises she created on particular healing themes. We were encouraged to report our images without embellishment or commentary and to describe our emotional and sensory responses. Colette's observations and comments taught us to read the images as hieroglyphs or symbols of our inner wisdom that could act as guideposts for changing our lives.

Transformations in consciousness and an out-flowing of creativity occurred throughout these Group Imagery sessions. Works of art were birthed, talents discovered, careers changed, our well-being improved—and as Colette described, there were "jumps toward the direction of Spirit." My own creative juices began to flow like a torrent, and I produced two books and a number of articles that were published during that time.

This group process was evolutionary, even revolutionary. Needless to say, I incorporated it into my regular teaching programs and integrative healthcare practice in New York City. Students' awareness expanded as they unveiled outgrown beliefs, replacing them with new ones that enriched their lives. Patients in my clinical practice resolved issues and renewed their zest for life in a very few sessions.

Encouraged by the outcomes, I founded the American Institute for Mental Imagery (AIMI) in 1978 to train clinicians in *Imagination, Phenomenology, and Imagery.* This educational program is approved by the New York State Board of Regents and has graduated many clinicians. The same positive outcomes that occurred in my Group Imagery sessions are regularly reported by AIMI graduates in their private practices and in agencies and institutions where they work.

The imagery exercises in this book were shared by Colette: their arrangement comes from my intuitive understanding and experience with their effect. They represent a segment of my teaching from 1994-2002. During that time, my students Barbarah and Serge Fedoroff were in my Group Imagery classes, and Barbarah studied with Colette as part of a group I took to Jerusalem for fifteen days. Following Colette's practice, I dictated the exercises to students after each class. Barbarah recorded these exercises in a word processing program, which Serge formatted and managed, making it possible for the exercises to be shared.

That nine-year collection of more than 2,100 exercises is presented in these pages. It covers an incredible breadth and depth of personal possibilities for anyone wanting to discover the transformative potential of the exercises. Included are more than 40 themes to aid you in penetrating the depths of your being by gently peeling away layers of false beliefs, misperceptions, and hurtful physical and emotional experiences. Among the themes are *Deep Cleansing From Infancy, Introspection, Resurrection Of The Body, Quest For Hidden Meaning, Regaining Health And Wholeness,* and *Images Of The Heart.*

The beauty of Colette's imagery is that it is simple, powerful, and quick, with the exercises taking from seconds to a minute. The images you discover reveal both where you are now and what possibilities are available to you. At each step of your practice, you will make new personal discoveries and see behaviors in a new light, all of them steps in your discovery, growth, self-development, and transformation.

Colette was fluent in several languages, was an inspiring poet, and had keen insight into people and their responses. These combined skills are evident in the language and structuring of her imagery exercises. Like poetry, they do not necessarily follow the rules of logic. They nonetheless are effective at bringing you to your inner realm, the repository of wisdom imprinted in you at birth. This wisdom will surface as personal images showing your potential to become a unified being.

Gerald Epstein, M.D., Editor
Founder and Director, American Institute for Mental Imagery

EDITOR'S WELCOME
BARBARAH L. FEDOROFF

The Encyclopedia of Mental Imagery: Colette Aboulker-Muscat's 2,100 Visualization Exercises for Personal Development, Healing, and Self-Knowledge is an anthology of imagery created by Mme. Colette Aboulker-Muscat, which takes seekers on a personal pilgrimage of self-discovery. On this imaginal journey you'll spend a few minutes a day following Colette's imagery instructions that have drawn thousands to their inner wisdom and truth. You can begin your journey by doing a single imagery exercise each morning to set the tone for your day. Or you might select another practice described by Dr. Gerald Epstein in "Creating A Practice That Resonates With You."

My imaginal pilgrimage began in 1993 after attending a holistic health conference, where Dr. Epstein presented a workshop on angels. As the workshop ended, he held up a book he had written, *Studies in Non-Deterministic Psychology,* and offered the copy to any one of us. A throng moved forward and reaching up without seeing over the crowd, I felt the book in my hand. Since nothing happens by chance, I considered the book a clue to the next step on my spiritual journey and registered for a class at the American Institute of Mental Imagery (AIMI) Adult Education Center, founded by Dr. Epstein.

In the mid-1990's, on two occasions, Dr. Epstein brought a group of imagery students to Jerusalem to study with his teacher, Colette. In the summer of 1994, I joined the group going on this pilgrimage. What struck me when meeting Colette was the contrast of her white hair, loosely coiled on her head, to her vivid blue eyes that held the wisdom of her then 85 years. Her eyes held the liveliness and joy of an exuberant child - the depth of knowing what it is to experience the Divine. She was a formidable presence who encouraged students by being true to who she was.

Colette's home had an intimate front garden separated from the street above by a blue gate. She told us this gate represented a threshold students crossed to acquire knowledge they then took with them as they left through the same gate. Most evenings, Colette entertained us in this garden with unusual games that revealed why each of us was there. These revelations were more surprising to us than to Colette, who could read someone in a flash.

During the day, our imagery sessions were held in a shaded sitting room decorated with family treasures and mounds of richly colored pillows. Most of the room was reserved for the many students who came from far and near to uncover their inherent wisdom hidden beneath their false beliefs.

In the spiritual richness of Jerusalem's Old City and Colette's sessions, I came to understand imagery as a prayer connecting us with the Divine.

As that understanding took root, I had an image of myself standing before a field of daisies with smiling, childlike faces. These occurrences shifted my understanding of work to that of a vocation to improve the early education of children. At the time, I was CEO of Programs for Parents (PfP), a company helping parents find childcare. As advocates, PfP influenced mandatory regulations for in-home care — and wrote the provisions for free childcare that became part of the federal welfare reform law, ensuring that participants have the support they need to complete job training and enter the workforce.

When I returned home, I shared my experiences with staff members, and a weekly group of voluntary imagers evolved. As we progressed, a group energy developed to pursue the intention of making quality childcare affordable to all families. We focused our imagery to do so by securing a state contract to coordinate childcare in our county, which was to include administering childcare subsidies based on income. Each morning several of us imaged ourselves casting a golden net over the county, drawing in the contract.

That image became a waking-life reality, and eventually we were awarded a state contract that annually subsidizes childcare for more than eight thousand children while their mothers work full-time jobs. With a focus on school readiness by kindergarten, the contract also provides training for childcare workers in targeted areas and rigorous standards for early learning programs. Children who attend these programs are achieving at levels competitive with school districts across the country, according to recent evaluations of third graders.

Since my early image of the field of daisies, PfP has served over 100,000 children. These achievements were acknowledged by a Resolution of the Joint Legislature of the State of New Jersey on October 28, 2009.

That work is behind me now. As I waited for whatever would unfold, I was invited by AIMI to use my imagery notes and to edit this book. The daisy image I had in Jerusalem is going through another cycle, this time for readers, like you, who are invited to renew your lives using Colette's work.

Embedded in Colette's imagery are universal truths taught through the ages by master teachers of many traditions and disciplines. Her genius is in weaving these ancient revelations into thousands of evocative imagery exercises. With few exceptions, the exercises are in Colette's exact words – poetic, precise, and concise if not always typical of American speech patterns. Once you start this practice, you'll become at ease with her unique style.

May your personal pilgrimage lead you to wisdom and truth.

Barbarah L. Fedoroff, Editor
Graduate, American Institute for Mental Imagery, Interfaith Minister

About Colette Aboulker-Muscat

"I have always been in the service of clarity. To find the peace of the depths, the pillar of light that created it had to go through the darkness and the transparent glassy greenness of the ocean."

Colette, in her autobiography,
La Vie N'est Pas Un Roman (Life Is Not a Novel)

In a life filled with extraordinary events, Colette's childhood was marked by her early awareness of spirit and the realization of the existence and healing power of inner illuminative experience. One of the unique qualities of Colette's imagery is its capacity to move us toward our inner spark of (Divine) light and truth so we may discover how to live each moment freely.

Colette was born into an aristocratic, kabbalistic Jewish family in Algeria in 1909. At four, she was diagnosed with an illness that required her silence for two weeks lest she seriously damage her vocal chords. That silence extended over three years through circumstances and a serious illness. In the silence, she learned to observe people and attune to her inner life. In her autobiography, Colette recounts a dream she had while battling scarlet fever. "Three nights in a row I dream I am the failing light… covered with thicker clouds until I myself become a cloud. When I wake up, I change my dream. I see myself all shining with the midday sun…The cloud arrives… but I blow it away…The cloud disappears or becomes a star. I have had the strength to do that for a whole week. Doctor says I am progressing."

Her healing wisdom, obvious at that young age, was carried down from her North African Kabbalist ancestors and was encouraged by her grandmother, who also was a healer. Her ancestral gifts, the family's commitment to service, and the discipline of her early silence all enriched the mosaic that was to become the Waking Dream and Group Imagery methods she later developed as part of her spiritual teaching and healing work.

When Colette was twelve years old, her father, a renowned neurosurgeon, allowed her to accompany him to the hospital where he was treating soldiers from World War I, assumed to be hopeless. Her gift of listening brought many soldiers comfort and, as she quietly observed them, she created mental imagery exercises to help heal them or assist them to pass peacefully.

Later, Colette studied psychology at the Sorbonne where she met Robert DeSoille, who developed an imaginal process called the "Directed Day Dream." As part of her Sorbonne training, she had to see him as a supervisor. His method differed markedly from hers, but they developed a friendly working relationship while she was a student. During this time, she continued her healing work with all who sought her help, a generous gift she extended throughout her life. Among the many illnesses she addressed were possession, in which she exorcised people of demons so they could regain their health, and cancer, which was encroaching on the lives of hundreds who reached out to her.

In 1954, Colette left the security of family and moved to Jerusalem. Thousands from around the world journeyed there to heal or to learn her Waking Dream and Group Imagery methods fashioned after the work of the ancient biblical prophets. She continued this work for nearly fifty years and was often seen sitting in the garden entrance to her home, where all were welcomed.

Part of Colette's legacy is this *Encyclopedia* as well as *Alone with the One,* a book of poetry; *Mea Culpa: Tales of Resurrection,* a collection of cases of possession; and thousands of unique and life-changing Imagery exercises. The poetry at the head of each imagery section comes from Colette's book, *Alone With The One.*

An Introduction to Mental Imagery

Simply put, imagery is the mind speaking to us in pictures. Like English, it is a language; but a *picture* language rather than a *word* language. Imagery conveys the higher wisdom of our minds and longing of our hearts. It is also how the mind "speaks" or instructs the body, so it is a natural healing modality. The imaginal experience comprises what we see, sense, feel, live and know. You may *see* images in color, black or white or shades of tone. Concurrently you may *feel* emotions such as joy or sadness, love or anger, etc. Likewise, you may physically *sense* in your body tingling, a rush of energy, constriction or relaxation of muscles, etc. Occasionally, you may hear sounds as well. In sum, imagery is the natural and true language of our inner life. Colette was a master of this language and taught people to quickly become their own masters as well. As she summed it up in her book *Mea Culpa* "the image is life, which comes to help life, and is the movement of life, that starts life moving again."

Inspiration and intuition are similar to imagery in as they too convey our higher wisdom. Consider when you suddenly are motivated to create something - ideas flow and you feel exuberant and joyful. This is called inspiration. Or "out of the blue" you have a solution to a problem that seemed to have no answer. This kind of thought is called intuition – information and knowledge that is revealed to you outside the rules of logic and reason. We experience the language of images in our dreams as well. Inspiration, intuition and dreams usually occur spontaneously, without our direct initiation. In the imagery process, images are likewise *received* rather then sought or conjured.

My experience with Colette revealed to me that imagery takes place in an inner realm of existence, free of time and space, where we access a "vertical axis" beyond the constraints of gravity. Spiritual seekers have acknowledged the existence of this vertical axis for centuries, and it is understood through all cultures as the axis of freedom.

Imagery always attempts to put us in connection with this vertical axis enabling us to escape the ordinary limitations of earth-bound living. In practicing this work, you may regularly find yourself on the vertical axis. Here's an example of making this connection:

A friend called and explained that he had viral conjunctivitis. I suggested that he imaginally take his eyes out of their sockets, wash them in healing waters, and put blue light in the sockets. Several days later, he reported that his eyes had begun improving once he started the exercise. He also noted that after he returned his eyes to the blue-light-filled sockets, the dark-green lush vegetation around the healing waters had burst into flowers. But why, he asked, did he always find himself moving upward to get to the healing waters. I explained that moving upward was the direction of freedom and healing. My friend had discovered what we call the vertical axis. Given my experience with imagery, it did not surprise me to learn, as I studied other healing systems, that all cultures and traditions have linked upward movement with transcendence, myths of flight, severing the bonds and limitations of everyday habitual behavior and activity, and finding new paths, new ways of being.

Your Guide to Doing Imagery

Colette's imagery holds transformative possibilities whether done sporadically to correct difficult life situations or during periods when you feel impelled to discover more about yourself. You can support these quests for self-discovery by tapping into your inner wisdom with a daily *Personal Imagery Practice*. However you incorporate imagery into your life, you'll soon feel at ease with the process. Let go of any preconceived ideas about the images you find. Whatever appears is correct and useful, even if it seems silly, enigmatic or impossible. As imagery is not bound by the laws of logic, anything is possible.

CREATING AN IMAGERY PRACTICE THAT RESONATES WITH YOU

The Encyclopedia is organized in healing **themes** such as Personal Restoration, Clarity, and Coming to Order. Each theme is composed of several **subheadings** that contain related exercises. For example, under the **theme** of Personal Restoration there are seven **subheadings.** These sub-headings include Self-Healing, Self-Sculpture and The Whole Person, to name a few.

To help you get started, here are three possible approaches to use this book. Select the one that appeals to you now and try it for a week. After that, you may try another if you wish. The aim is to find an approach that supports the development of your Personal Imagery Practice.

1) Spontaneous Selection: *Spontaneously* open the book to a page and start at the beginning of that theme. This approach is often helpful to address an individual situation you'd like to change, but can be used as a regular practice as well. When you have completed the theme, you may continue with this spontaneous selection process.

2) Personal Appeal or Circumstance: Scan through the *Table of Contents* and select a theme that appeals to you or pertains to a current life situation. When you complete the theme, select another meaningful theme.

3) Following The Book: Begin with the first theme in the book. When you complete it, move on, following each theme in order.

AUDIO RECORD THE EXERCISES

With the ready availability of miniature recording devices built into smart phones, you may prefer to audio record your selection of exercises and then playback the recording for your imagery practice; alternatively, you can read each exercise individually, and then do it imaginally; or possibly enlist someone to read the imagery to you as you do it. Of course, you can always organize a group imagery session.

Instructions for Imaging

Imagery succeeds in direct proportion to our success in turning our senses away from the stimulation of the outside world to a calm, inner realm. As discussed below there are three simple steps to begin imaging: sit upright in a chair, close your eyes, and breathe out. (Note: In several of my other books on mental imagery, I discuss setting an intention. With this work, it is unnecessary.)

HOW TO SIT FOR IMAGERY

The most effective body position for imaging is to sit in what I call the "Pharaoh's Posture." Throughout the ages, royalty assumed this posture seeking inner guidance before making a decision. *It is a posture expressing awareness, wakefulness, strength, and independence.*

In the Pharaoh's posture, you sit upright in a straight-backed chair that has arms. Keeping your back straight, rest your arms comfortably on the armrests, your hands open, palms down. (If you have no armrests, just put your hands in your lap). Place your feet flat on the floor. Try not to cross your hands or your feet or touch other parts of your body while you image. This helps keep your sensory awareness focused inward, away from external stimuli.

While the Pharaoh's Posture is ideally suited to imaging, there are instances in which an imagery exercise has to be done instantly; for example, when you are experiencing anxiety. In these situations, you can image standing up, even with your eyes open, wherever you are.

CLOSE YOUR EYES TO TURN INWARD

In imagery, we generally keep our eyes closed to shut out external diversions and distractions. If you are uncomfortable with this, keep your eyes open. At the end of an exercise, or at the end of several short exercises, you open your eyes briefly before starting the next exercise.

HOW TO BREATHE FOR IMAGERY:
OUTBREATH/INBREATH

To help direct our attention inward and induce a light relaxation, we start by breathing *out* a long, slow exhalation through the *mouth,* and follow it with a normal inhalation through the *nose*, i.e., don't exaggerate the *in*breath. Do this **three (3)** times - an exhalation followed by an inhalation, an exhalation followed by an inhalation, and an exhalation followed by an inhalation. This is noted in the text as **BO3X,** short for *breathe out three times.* Once you complete this cycle, your breathing can resume its natural pattern. During imagery work, your attention will be focused on the images and your breathing will take care of itself.

At the end of an exercise or imagery set take **one** *out*breath before you open your eyes. This induces an inner calm and will bring you back to everyday life in a quiet, centered way.

As you go through the Encyclopedia, you will see variations on this basic breathing technique. For example, sometimes an imagery exercise may instruct you to start by taking a single *out*breath, noted as **BO1X,** short for *breathe out one time*; or two rounds, noted as **BO2X** (short for *breathe out two times)*. Occasionally, there may be different breathing instructions that are fully noted in the text. **And of course, if you forget to follow a breathing instruction exactly, just proceed with the exercise.** After a few imagery exercises, the varied breathing instructions will become second nature. You can find a short video on this breathing at my website: *http:// drjerryepstein.org/encyclopedia/breathing*

UNDERSTANDING THE ICONS
BETWEEN EXERCISES

You'll notice there are icons ( ) between many of the exercises. They provide a brief rest between exercises. Taken together the three icons instruct you to: **Breathe out (** **), open your eyes (** **),** rest a moment, then **close your eyes (** **)** before beginning the next exercise. If there are no icons between exercises, just keep your eyes closed. These icons are also used at the start of a group of exersices to remind you to close your eyes **(** **)** and at the completion of a group of exercises to remind you to breath out and open your eyes **(** **).**

IN IMAGERY, LESS IS MORE

Many of us tend to think that more effort brings greater results, but imagery works in the opposite way. Paradoxically, the shorter the time you stay in an image, the more powerful the result will be. Most imagery exercises are short and take only 5 to 15 seconds - or occasionally up to a minute to complete. If you don't relate to an exercise or respond to it after several seconds, just breathe out once, open your eyes, and move on to the next image.

IF AT FIRST YOU CAN'T IMAGE

Not everyone has the same capacity for imaging. For most, the process comes easily, almost at once. Others may need more practice before imaging comes to them. Here are a few tips to stimulate your capacity for imaging:

Look at pictures or photographs of natural settings for 20-30 seconds, then close your eyes and see the same pictures appear in your mind. Another approach is to remember a pleasant scene from your past, with your eyes open. Then close your eyes and remember these images. You can also use your non-visual senses. For example, hear fish frying in a skillet or the applause of an audience or glasses clinking; or smell perfumes or essences of varying strengths and experience what happens.

You can also practice relying first on the senses you use or respond to most easily. For example, if you're an auditory person, hear the sound of the ocean and sense what images emerge. When you consciously focus your attention on what you are sensing, they can convert spontaneously into other sensory experiences. Remember that our senses turned inward allow us to discover this inner realm of self-awareness, self-knowledge, self-wisdom and self-understanding. In this regard imagination is recognized as the inner super-sensory organ of perception, an inner light guiding our senses to make these discoveries.

Some people have the habit of verbalizing rather than visualizing, turning images quickly into words. If this applies to you, practice looking around at your environment for a few minutes without naming, labeling, or categorizing what you see. If you reflexively start to name things, just return to the practice of seeing without further elaboration. Over time, you will find the imagery emerge more and more spontaneously.

ESTABLISHING A DAILY IMAGERY PRACTICE

Plan to spend a few minutes each day practicing imagery. Generally, you will do each set of exercise only once, moving on to another set the following day. If you have a strong response to an exercise or series of exercises, take a moment after you complete the exercise(s) to jot it down along with your responses. Writing down the imagery anchors it in consciousness. If you wish, you may repeat the exercise(s) once a day in the morning for another six days before going on to a new selection.

You may find yourself spontaneously modifying exercises. Go right ahead. You are calling on yourself to participate in your growth and healing. Should you be left with an occasional image that is disturbing or distressing simply reverse or correct the image. Here are examples of how to correct an image: If you find yourself in a dark cave, light a torch or turn on a flashlight; if you find yourself in prison, find a golden key to unlock the door.; if you cannot see something clearly, use a golden magnifying glass; if you feel a cramp, imaginally see your muscles elongating. Remember, this is imagination - anything can happen!

TIMES OF DAY TO PRACTICE IMAGERY

If possible schedule your Personal Imagery Practice before starting your daily routine - that is, before breakfast, enabling you to start your day in a new way. Otherwise, do it at twilight, and/or at the end of the day before bed. Together, these three times are natural prayer and mediation times, potent transition points when information from other realms is more readily accessible. Be consistent in your practice. This really cannot be emphasized enough. Not compulsive, just consistent.

GLOSSARY OF UNFAMILIAR WORDS

Words that are unfamiliar are followed by an asterisk (*). Definitions for these words can be found in the glossary at the back of the book.

CREATING YOUR PERSONAL IMAGERY SPACE

If possible, reserve a space in your home where you can be alone and without interruptions. Set the space up with:

- ► A comfortable, straight-back armchair;
- ► Natural lighting if possible;
- ► A notebook and pens to jot down exercises;
- ► A recorder to pre-record your selected exercises, if you wish.

A CHECKLIST FOR GETTING STARTED

► Pick an approach to use this book selecting your first theme, exercise set or single exercise. If you prefer, you can audio record the exercises in advance.

► Sit upright in the Pharaoh's Posture, close your eyes (▧), and take a long, slow exhalation (*out*breath) followed by a brief or normal inhalation (*in*breath). Do this a total of three times **(BO3X).** Thereafter, breathe in any way that is comfortable for you, allowing the imagery to form in your consciousness.

► Complete one or more exercises. Between exercises, follow the icons - *breathe out* (◉), *open your eyes* (◎) *& close your eyes* (▧). Conclude your last imagery exercise each day by *breathing out one time and opening your eyes* (◉◎). If you become tired at any point, stop! breathe out and open your eyes – you have had enough imagery for the day.

There's only one thing left to do. Begin imaging. Bon voyage!

Personal Restoration

"I am not part of Totality! Totality is me, into me.
I know then that I am infinite, immortal. New Forever."
—Colette, "Knowing"

SELF-HEALING

BO3X ▸ COUNTING SILENTLY FROM 3 TO 1, EACH OUT-BREATH BEING A NEW NUMBER. See the "1" as a lighthouse sending you light to make you more lucid and to make what you do, perfectly clear.

SELF-SCULPTURE

BO3X ▸ Hold a double handful of clay. Get acquainted with the clay. Feel its texture and weight and the way it changes shape as you explore it with your fingers by pushing, shaking, pinching. Discover what this clay is like as you shape it by squeezing, patting, and pulling, and discover what it is capable of.

BO3X ▸ Now shape all the clay into a ball and focus your awareness in your hands and fingers that have just been exploring the clay. Notice how your fingers feel. Now turn inward and focus on different areas of your body. Become aware of what you feel in each different area. Now visualize an image of your round ball of clay and imagine it changing slowly into an image of yourself. It may become an abstract of you, or a clear image. Whatever it does, watch it closely as it develops without interference from you.

BO3X ▸ Focus your attention on your hands and fingers as they move and get acquainted with the clay again. Now create an image of yourself feeling the clay with your fingers and using your fingers to create your shape. See what develops out of the process of shaping yourself out of the clay.

THE WHOLE PERSON ► SEXUALITY:
FOR IMPOTENCE AND FRIGIDITY

BO3X ► See, feel, and know your own individual, personal energetic dimension.

BO1X ► Feel and sense how it is made by needs, dreams and passions.

BO1X ► See how by choosing or not, you are involved in familial, social, and political dynamics.

BO1X ► Feel and sense how the energy coming from your sexuality may be a reinforcement of all your life.

BO3X ► See and know how you are feeling as a man, as a provider, as a husband and an aggressor and as a woman, a receiver, a nurturer, a mother and wife.

BO3X ► See and know how love, monogamy, respect, and sexual privacy are protecting and strengthening the human condition.

BX3X ► Sense and feel how sexuality is a charging, thrilling, playful thing. When exchanged freely and experimented or experienced with others, it becomes a tool for traveling to new regions and for entering our own self-exploring adventures.

BO3X ► Know how it makes us free to examine our minds, our feelings, our bodies, and the dynamics of the sexuality itself.

BO3X ► See and feel how long relationships encourage deep connections. See how some brief relationships may offer a closeness no others permit because they are free from expectation, inhibition, history, agenda, and free of all that places conditions on long relationships.

BO3X ► See and know if you are ready to sacrifice long-term commitment and stability for short-term intensity, variety, excitement, and freedom of movement.

BO3X ► See and know the possible reasons why we join with another person:

BO1X ► For energetic release;

BO1X ► For emotional support;

BO1X ► For sheer sensory delight;

BO1X ► For the opportunity of personal growth;

BO1X ► For psychic interchange;

BO1X ► For egotistical challenge;

BO1X ► For spiritual enhancement or encounter.

BO1X ► See each of these as a way of communicating your deep love and as a struggle for clarity.

BO3X ► See how improving health, heightening the quality of life, and expanding awareness comes from permitting ourselves the birth of new myths. At first, these myths are related to our personal body, mind, health, and self-development and later to our social and cultural behavior. Note your feelings about this.

BO3X ► Know how the slightest form of pride prevents you from knowing the truth.

BO3X ► Know how unless there is truth in you, there can be no falsehood in others.

BO3X ► See and feel some great difficulties.

BO3X ► Live overcoming these difficulties as a great adventure.

....

THE WORK OF INNER JOURNEY

BO3X ► Live some self-denial as delayed gratification. Know why denial pays off.

BO3X ► Know how the impulse of self-fulfillment makes for restless searching and spending.

BO3X ► See and know how self-fulfillment is asking for freedom and is pushing us to avoid lifestyles.

BO1X ► Know that when freedom is preserved for us, we ask what to do with it.

BO3X ▸ Feel and know how in going to extremes, we become self-absorbed and preoccupied with the self.

BO1X ▸ See and feel the difference between search and self-indulgence when involved with the self.

BO3X ▸ See and live the difference between introspection and the search for the awareness for meaning.

BO3X ▸ Know and see how the restless seekers have permitted gurus to make false promises that they will bring us out of the darkness into the light.

....

BEING OR NOT BEING: FOR MINDBODY HEALTH AND SELF DEVELOPMENT

BO3X ▸ Feel in yourself the tension between stability and change.

BO1X ▸ Feel and know the powerful drive to maintain the sense of your identity for continuity.

BO1X ▸ See and recognize some fear of changing too fast or of being changed by outside forces.

BO3X ▸ Feel and recognize your powerful, striving organism and your desire to be more than you are now.

BO3X ▸ See and know that to fulfill your possibilities you have to exchange your self-esteem and your sense of control over your life for ultimate values.

BO3X ▸ See, feel, and know if all along in your life you have had some stable qualities, like being gregarious and assertive or if all along in your life you have had the qualities of being introverted and anxious or if you have had the constant quality of being impulsive.

BO3X ▸ Feel and know if these constant traits are inherited, biological disposi-tions, influences from childhood, or patterns of social roles and expectations.

BO1X ▸ See and know which of these traits you are locked into.

BO3X ▸ Know and feel how change cannot be accomplished if you are denying.

BO1X ▸ Know and feel how change cannot be accomplished if you are denying the existence and rights of another. Feel how this denial is blind and wrong.

BO3X ▸ See how you have created a situation concerning denial offering you the chance to reform and change.

BO3X ▸ When feeling empty or sad because you have to cut with a preceding part of life you have loved or liked, join your two hands on your heart and entwine your fingers. Capture your feeling and throw it away, smiling all the time as you renounce and remove the feeling so you are free to live a new life.

BO3X ▸ See yourself changing by the Eight-fold Path of the Buddha.

BO1X ▸ See right views that bring right understanding.

BO1X ▸ See right purpose that brings right intention or aspiration.

BO1X ▸ See right speech that brings you to a right way of life.

BO1X ▸ See right conduct that brings you to a right way of life.

BO1X ▸ See right livelihood that brings you to a right way of life.

BO1X ▸ See right effort that brings you to a right way of life.

BO1X ▸ See the right kind of awareness or mindfulness needed now.

BO1X ▸ See the right concentration or meditation needed now.

BO3X ▸ See and know how we are witnessing a moment of cosmic truth.

EVOLUTION OF HUMOR:
TO BECOME PSYCHOLOGICALLY SOUND

"A joyous spirit avoids and heals all suffering."
- Mindest

BO2X ► Look at some situation. Feel and recognize your sense of ineptitude and inadequacy. Laugh to tears.

BO3X ► See and feel how when becoming aggressive and sexual, you are directing hostility and ridicule toward others.

BO3X ► Feel and sense your humor and your ability to laugh at personal shortcomings. Do it in a confident, non-threatening manner.

BO3X ► Feel and live how this confident way is bringing effective control over your life.

BO3X ► Feel and know the seriousness of humor.

BO1X ► Live and know how humor is helping you develop self-esteem and self-worth.

BO3X ► Live and know how humor helps you to develop social interests and real interest in others.

BO1X ► Live and recognize how self-worth and interest in others are necessary qualities over which you may have absolute self-control.

BO1X ► Know how by using humor you can make these qualities fully operational.

BO3X ► Imagine you and others in a situation where you are laughing.

BO1X ► Who is laughing most in the situation? (If not you, continue the exercise).

BO1X ► How can you participate more fully in the laughter?

BO3X ► What do you see to be the most funny? What is causing the laughter?

BO1X ► How can the situation become funnier for you and for others? Are you enjoying the laughter?

BO1X ► Do or say something funny for the situation.

BO3X ► Feel yourself not undignified or irreverent, but more candid, more perceptive, and more fully self-accepting.

SEXOLOGY ► SURVIVAL OF THE HUMAN SPECIES: FOR RESOLVING RELATIONSHIPS

BO3X ► See and live how our character is opposed to or hidden by what we are saying. Recognize the character of your behavior. [Character is the tool inscribing what we are].

BO1X ► Feel and be aware of how you speak, knowing how the voice is a secondary sexual organ. Pay attention not to push the one you are talking to against the wall of negativity.

To Life: To Live

"I change all the time. And you change also. Every thing existing is changing too and we depend on each other."
-Colette, "Creation"

SYMBOLISM

BO3X ▸ COUNTING SILENTLY FROM 3 TO 1, EACH OUT-BREATH BEING A NEW NUMBER. Imagine yourself looking into a mirror. See how going backwards and upside-down is changing all your old habits and cleaning you out.

BO3X ▸ COUNTING SILENTLY FROM 3 TO 1, EACH OUT-BREATH BEING A NEW NUMBER. Imagine yourself becoming the number one. See and live how diabolic is the opposite of symbolic and therefore brings disunion.

BO3X ▸ COUNTING SILENTLY FROM 3 TO 1, EACH OUT-BREATH BEING A NEW NUMBER. Imagine yourself looking into a mirror. See and know how a symbol is an image of that which has been cut in two, becomes diabolical, and how reorganization occurs when the two parts are put together.

BO3X ▸ See yourself writing into the mirror a diabolical word. See how it is a perverted symbol, reappearing in waking life as a symptom.

BO3X ▸ Know how the fault in the origin of the symptom is feelings of guilt. See how we use our symbol to vanquish a diabolic word or a perverted symbol.

SELF IMAGE ▸ PERSONAL IDENTITY

BO3X ▸ See yourself right now, then BO1X and see your image in a mirror. Look at this image receding farther and farther from you and reconstruct it piece-by-piece as your guide, your angel keeper, or your wise advisor. Ask this helpmate for advice.

BO3X ▸ You have a multi-faceted mirror with 12 facets and one center. Look at each facet of the mirror one-by-one, seeing in each, a direction your life has taken. When you have lived each of these images of yourself, erase them by cleaning each facet of the mirror. Now you are at the central mirror. See yourself as you want to be with the experiences of your life.

IN KNOWN:
TO REVERSE EARLY DESTRUCTIVE CONDITIONING

BO4X ▸ Live in yourself these stages of development as an inner road that is oral, anal, phallic, and genital. See and live all their sensations and emotions.

BO2X ▸ Again, follow the inner road and feel the lingering energy in each of these stages and places.

BO3X ▸ Sense how these inside borders or frontiers are where mucous membranes and skin are meeting. Sense and feel how these places are as ocean shores or tides that the energy is lapping, beating, and caressing.

HEART CONSTRICTION

"Heart Constriction is a shock to the heart. People with weight in their stomach constrict their heart. They then experience things first in the neck and then below. Do an image to enlarge the larynx and throat muscles."
-Colette

BO3X ▸ See your larynx becoming very large and your throat muscles becoming very strong.

Deep Cleansing From Infancy

"Night and Day...
I am waiting for you to give the kiss of life."
-Colette, "The Kiss of Life"

DEEP CLEANSING FROM INFANCY:
TO REVERSE DESTRUCTIVE CONDITIONING

BO3X ▸ Watch carefully for the strategies you use to maintain your alien identity. This identity was conferred on you in your formative years, beginning at age four.

BO1X ▸ Do you feel imprisoned by these strategies? Trapped? How do you feel now?

BO1X ▸ Ask yourself why you recall these particular scenes.

BO1X ▸ Know what has made you the person you are now.

BO1X ▸ What are the two most significant events in your life?

BO1X ▸ Allow your images to reveal you as you have been in the past and as you are now.

BO3X ▸ Return now to your childhood at ages 4 or 5. Imagine the emotions you felt and the places, events, and people connected with these emotions. With your hand, wash away or brush away the emotions that are distressing to you to the left.

BO1X ▸ See, sense, and feel how all the exercises have affected you. Give yourself a numerical mark between 1 for slightly effected and 20 for greatly effected.

....

CLEARING WITH TEARS

BO3X ▸ See your tears being cleared by the sun and see a white cloud being formed. Then see a drop of water being dropped on the cloud and watch the cloud becoming a lake of tears. See this lake being absorbed by the sun.

ANGELS' MEDITATION: FOR SELF KNOWING

BO3X ▸ Imagine God's palaces and the Guardian Angels at the threshold of each chamber. See seven palaces each with ten chambers. At each threshold, look directly into the eyes of the Guardian Angel and see what you have to face and learn there.

CYCLES OF LIFE

BO3X ▸ Sense and know how in getting our body from God and our parents, we don't dare let it be destroyed.

BO1X ▸ Feel yourself as the master of your body and of your mind.

BO1X ▸ See how you have become the master.

BO1X ▸ See yourself falling into depression or sadness.

BO1X ▸ See yourself light with gladness.

BO1X ▸ Know how it is up to you to change and choose your attitude.

BO3X ▸ Live and know what life and death are.

BO1X ▸ Live them now, seeing yourself casting out frustration, resentment, blame, guilt, doubt, disease, aging, death.

BO3X ▸ See yourself as a newborn, as an infant, as a child. Have all their feelings.

BO3X ▸ See yourself as an adult, as an old one. Have all their sensations, ideas, and feelings.

BO3X ▸ See yourself as a dead one, as a newborn. Now live, renewed with aliveness.

REPENTANCE*:
REVERSING ERRORS OF THE PAST

BO3X ► See yourself traveling on the back of a dragon. See how you are climbing with it through all the stages of development by flying from inside of the earth to the highest mountain and from cloud to cloud above the 7 skies and return.

BO3X ► See and sense the Archangel Raphael* standing behind you.

BO1X ► Do a reversing examination of consciousness beginning now and going backwards to your earliest childhood. See how doing this helps you recognize every pain you have caused others and yourself.

BO1X ► Repair every damage you have done to others. See yourself asking for forgiveness from those you have offended, humiliated, or abused.

BO1X ► Discover the guilts that bring you feelings of shame and regret. Know how by keeping them alive, you allow them to take too much space in you.

BO3X ► Repent at every moment the evil done in the past beginning from now back to your conception.

BO1X ► Repent honestly with all your heart.

BO1X ► Sense the new well-being filling you when repenting as you return from the time of conception to now, coming back cleansed.

BO3X ► When at the peak of repenting, you are reaching the now. Feel you are no longer blaming others or yourself. See a river flowing through you, cleansing you.

....

CLEANSING YOUR SOUL ►
THE LIGHT BEARING SOUL

BO3X ► Imagine a lake in the sky. See that it is a lake of tears.

BO1X ► Imagine pain or difficulty leaving you as a flaming ball falling into the lake of tears.

BO1X ► A drop of water falls from above onto the lake of tears and becomes part of this lake in the sky.

BO1X ▶ See and know what the flaming ball becomes when it falls into the lake in the sky.

BO1X ▶ See your soul going out of you to hunt the sky for the ball of fire. Face your soul when it comes out of the lake in the sky.

BO1X ▶ See and sense what is happening and have your soul re-enter you.

AGAINST ANXIETY

Note: "Anxiety only occurs in linear time. There is always a story called 'second voice'. Anxiety is torment and twisting. It is first mental and then it is reflected physically. It brings a fear of mental illness. Women especially are alerted not to torment or be tormented. See yourself worrying about the future and you will see how your torment increases. Fundamental anxiety can happen in the birthing through tension in the neck as it elongates." – Colette

"Anguish is a physical, agonizing pain. It is battling with pain and it is better to surrender to it." -Colette

BO3X ▶ BREATHING OUT THE TOXINS OF ANGST* — Experience the physical narrowing that occurs when being tied up or constricted.

BO3X ▶ Sense yourself being tied up, especially aware of your throat. Sense the angst inside yourself.

AGAINST ANGUISH

BO3X ▶ Sense anguish in your body. See yourself vanquishing pain in a battle.

BO3X ▶ Imagine a spike or long nail in your flesh. What do you feel?

BO3X ► Imagine you are visiting the four corners of your bedroom. What do you find? What do you ignore?

BO3X ► Imagine you have a watch in which there is a wheel that is not perfect.

BO1X ► Open the watch, clean the dust off each piece, and repair the damaged wheel.

BO1X ► Put everything back in place in the correct order, and now that it is repaired, hear what the watch is telling you.

HEADACHES, BACK PAIN

BO3X ► See a big, gold chain with huge links. Put it at your first vertebrae down to the tailbone, not touching your body. Take it down the back of your legs, slowly, placing it behind your feet. What do you feel in your feet?

PRAYER FOR WHEN NOT FEELING WELL

BO3X, CHANT THE HEBREW WORD RAFUAH*, PRONOUNCED IN ENGLISH AS RA-FOO-AH, TO THE MUSICAL NOTES MI-DO-RE (E, C AND D) OUT LOUD, THREE TIMES.

Then, see yourself in a dark forest moving toward a distant light. Find yourself in a clearing. In the clearing, a light from above is creating a circle on the ground. Stand in that circle of light and say a short healing prayer ending with "Thy Will Be Done." See yourself taken up into the hands of God.

HEALING BY REFUSING GUILT AND EVIL

BO3X ► Looking into a mirror, see evil and guilt. See yourself refusing evil and guilt.

BO1X ► Clean out the mirror to the left, using your left hand.

BO1X ▸ Turn over the mirror to its other face and see what good is appearing in place of the evil and guilt. Rest with this good, becoming assured of its eventual perfect accomplishment. See it done.

BO1X ▸ See yourself climbing a very high ladder to see behind the clouds. What do you see?

BO1X ▸ From behind the clouds, what do you feel? If you feel guilt, what is the guilt about?

BO1X ▸ Know the standard of guilt to which you respond.

BO1X ▸ See how you fight only yourself when you make the world your adversary.

BO1X ▸ See your error in this behavior.

ILLUSIONS: FROM RICHARD BACH*

BO3X ▸ See how the depth of your belief in injustice and tragedy may be the mark of ignorance.

BO1X ▸ See yourself not isolated but a part of the whole.

BO1X ▸ Keep in mind only images of health, kindness, goodness, and love.

BO1X ▸ Sense and see their abundance.

SHOOTING THE ARROW TO REACH A GOAL

THIS IS A POWERFUL EXERCISE TO BE DONE ONLY ONCE A YEAR.

BO3X ▸ Stand in an open space. See yourself with a bow and arrow. The bow is made of wood and gold. Stand straight, with your feet firmly on the ground, and bring the bow and arrow to your third eye*. Hear its sound. Bring it to eye level and hear its sound. Bring it to ear level and hear its sound. Feel your feet, your legs, your chest, your arms, your head, your connection with your target. Close your eyes, pull back the arrow and bowstring and let the arrow go, knowing it will reach the target.

BO3X ▸ See a 7-year-old boy standing in a clearing with a bow and arrow. See him shooting the arrow at a star and having it come back to his heart. What happens?

TRANSMISSIONS OF GRACE

WITH YOUR EYES OPEN BO3X AND THEN LOOK AT A SPOT ON THE CEILING.

BO3X ▸ AND THEN IMAGINALLY DRAW A SIX-POINTED STAR AROUND THE SPOT.

WITH YOUR EYES OPEN, BO1X SLOWLY AND THEN SOUND THE NAME E-LI-JAH SIX TIMES SILENTLY TO THE MUSICAL NOTES OF MI, DO, RE (E,C,D).

BO3X ▸ Sense the hands of Elijah* upon your hands as you imaginally look down on a duplicate of yourself stretched out on a bed.

BO1X ▸ See your palms together, and direct them toward your resting body. Move them horizontally from your eyes to your toes in slow rhythmic movements.

BO1X ▸ At the same time, sense Elijah blowing upon both the standing and the resting you.

BO1X ▸ Hear yourself breathing your name.

BO1X ▸ Look at the star you have drawn on the ceiling and see its radiant rays touching the resting you at the points where a healing is necessary.

BO3X ▸ Know and feel how what you accept is delivered to you by your all-knowing mind.

BO1X ▸ See, observe, and accept only what you decide is good for you and not harmful to others.

SYMPTOMS ▸ MESSAGES OF THE FACE:
FOR EARLY SYMPTOMS OF DISTRESS

BO3X ▸ Become aware of the strong part of your face.

BO3X ▸ Become aware of the weak part of your face.

BO3X ► Have the strong part of your face speak to the weak part.

BO3X ► Have the weak part of your face make a statement to the strong part of your face. How is your face now? Make any repairs needed.

....

SYMPTOMS ► MESSAGES OF THE HANDS: FOR EARLY SYMPTOMS OF DISTRESS

PLACE YOUR HANDS ON YOUR LAP THROUGHOUT THIS EXERCISE.

BO3X ► With your hands on your lap, become aware of all the sensations coming from them.

BO1X ► Now become your right hand.

BO1X ► Now become your left hand.

BO3X ► Have your right hand saying something to your left hand.

BO3X ► Have your left hand saying something to your right hand.

BO1X ► Feel the interdependence of the two hands and sense how they cooperate.

BO3X ► Feel if there is some tension between your hands. Be aware that this tension may be creating symptoms or bad habits. Become conscious of these bad habits in your waking life.

BO3X ► Be aware of some physical symptom.

BO1X ► And increase the symptom. THEN OPEN YOUR EYES.

BO1X ▸ CLOSE YOUR EYES and diminish the symptom. Diminish the symptom even further either by letting go, forgetting, fighting, explaining it, or by choosing a way of your own.

BO3X ▸ See and know what your symptom is telling you and what message it gives others.

CLEARING THOUGHT AND EMOTION FROM THE BRAIN: FOR EARLY SYMPTOMS OF DISTRESS

BO3X ▸ See your hair growing long. Wash it with rum and egg yolks. Rinse it thoroughly with pure water, then lift off your skullcap, and look into your brain. Now turn the skullcap upside down and use your long hair to wash your brain. Rinse the brain with clear water that falls from a cloud in the sky. Put your skullcap back on and wash your hair again with egg yolks and rum, rinse your hair again with pure water, and see your hair returning to its regular length.

PRAYER: SILENCE

BO3X ▸ See, feel, and sense how the only praise worthy of God is silence.

BO3X ▸ See the likeness of the speaking silence. Know how by listening to the silence, you hear the life within you being the helper of your life and you hear this life within you being the helper of all life. OPEN YOUR EYES QUICKLY.

PRAYER OF RABBI NACHMAN OF BRESLOV*:
FOR DEPRESSION

"He was clinically depressed but lived in joy."
- Colette.

BO3X ▸ Keep Still.

BO1X ▸ Keep a reverent silence.

BO1X ▸ Feel and know how the reward for this silence is Divine Mercy that will not cease descending upon you.

BO3X ▸ See and live how this silent prayer is vibrating from world to world according to the spirit inhabiting it.

BO1X ▸ Follow the silent vibration of your prayer. Try to hear the silent words of wisdom contained in it for now and forever.

....

THE DIM LIGHT OF THE UNHEARD SOUND:
TO BECOME WHOLE

"Enthusiasm reflects the God within. Passion reflects passivity that draws."
- Colette.

BO3X ▸ Live the uncreated light of the beginning and of the end.

BO3X ▸ Once again, see and sense yourself attracted to the vibration of this light.

BO1X ▸ Feel yourself being taken into the light by the vibration of its tremendous sound.

BO1X ▸ Sense that the sound is coming out from the beginning and the end.

BO3X ▸ See and sense that in returning to the light and sound, we have returned to ourselves and are no more in exile on the earth.

BO3X ▸ See and sense like Abraham, that you are able to sacrifice the credibility and possibility of the past with its richness and beauty for the truth of now.

BO1X ▸ Feel and see that by this sacrifice, you are reintegrating the evident, ultimate light.

THE JUST SOUND

BO3X ▸ Feel, hear, and see how words, sounds, and rhythm are bringing a message. Feel and know how the right words and the right sounds are those that are in justice and harmony, and are bearing the message of being just and in harmony.

BO3X ▸ Feel and know how by listening to the sound of your just voice, you recognize that it brings justice with recourse and harmony.

BO1X ▸ Listen to the sound of your voice in enthusiasm and in passion and pay attention to the difference.

IDENTITY

BO3X ▸ Feel and know how your identity looks like a ladder of smaller selves.

BO3X ▸ Feel, see, and know how it is to be united with the Divine Soul at the top of the ladder.

BO3X ▸ Step onto the first rung of the ladder. Here live, sense, and know the excitement of taking this journey to the Divine Soul.

BO1X ▸ Moving up to the second rung, live your animal nature, experienced in sleep.

BO1X ▸ Live your way to spirit across your images, passing through your animal nature again.

BO3X ▸ Step up now to the third rung of the ladder. Stay on the third rung to receive information about the future. Know this information may be mixed up or distorted.

BO3X ▸ Step up now to the fourth rung of the ladder. Know your living essence by the purity of its purpose with real inspiration.

BO3X ▸ Step up now to the fifth rung of the ladder. Live union with the Unique Essence by cleaving to it. Sense your clear consciousness and calm feelings.

BO3X ▸ Feel and know how only by being undistracted from your path, are you elevating to perfect union with your Divine Essence.

BO3X ▸ See yourself as an old man heading toward a narrow bridge. Know that you must cross the bridge to the other side. As you walk across, the sea and the wind rise and the bridge sways from left to right. Halfway across, a monster rises from the water, then a devil with red eyes jumps in front of you. You know you must go beyond the devil to the other side. What happens? How do you feel?

···

TREE OF LIFE

BO3X ▸ See yourself as the Tree of Life, the Tree of Knowledge, the serpent, Eve and the apple. When you are all of these at the same moment, how do you feel?

BO3X ▸ You are standing at the edge of the Sea of Galilee. You sense a layer of energy beneath you. The wind surrounds you and you walk on the Sea of Galilee.

Wilhelm Reich* Imagery

"In the abyss of the unknown are hideous monsters...
Calm and quiet, I wait for those that are just there. Then they
transform into fresh charming youths, ready for the quest."
-Colette, "The Green Lion Swallows the Sun"

SURVIVAL OF THE HUMAN SPECIES ▶ SOCIETY'S NEUROSES

BO3X ▶ See how these resigned, impotent characters who have neuroses have strong underlying sadistic and rebellious impulses.

BO3X ▶ See and know how people with this structure are longing for freedom and independence, but are deeply afraid of it.

BO1X ▶ See and know how these people are becoming "one of the herd" as a bull or a stallion, castrated to make them docile.

BO3X ▶ See how such character structure on a mass scale has made people open to repressive and reactionary political movements that constantly undermine the best efforts toward democracy and real humanitarian reforms.

MINDSET

BO3X ▶ See and sense in yourself how the flu and colds are the releasing of suppressed emotion.

BO3X ▶ See and know how the blockage of energy in ourselves may be the root cause of war, racism, sexism, the exploitation of one group by another, fascism or dictatorships.

BO1X ▶ Know and feel how all of it is based on hatred.

BO3X ► Live chronic frustration. Establish the source of this disagreeableness.

BO3X ► See and feel how the authoritarian, anti-life attitudes of the masses reflect authoritarian, oppressive, family upbringing.

BO3X ► Live how this type of upbringing makes us impotent and resigns us to a life submissive to authority and lacking in genuine self-confidence.

SEXOLOGY: FOR OVERCOMING SEXUAL INHIBITIONS

BO3X ► Live and see how sensing perfect orgasm permits us to have a supply of energy we may use purposefully, when we don't search only for it.

BO3X ► Sense and feel how Reich wanted to cure neuroses by changing western feelings about sex.

BO1X ► Sense and feel how fearful attitudes about sex are connected with our actual feelings of disgrace, shame, and strategies of self-punishment.

BO3X ► Sense, live, and feel how resisting such a massive push of primal energy is changing the orgasm reflex to orgasm anxiety with bad feelings and arrhythmic contractions.

BO3X ► Sense and live completely the enormous build-up of energy followed by the releasing waves of our entire body musculature.

BO3X ► Feel and live the melting and streaming of a loss of egotism and the profound feelings of peace, fulfillment, and tenderness that come with the releasing waves of the body musculature. See the different colors connected with these sensations and feelings.

INTO THE MIRROR, SEE YOUR FACE:
TO REMOVE SYMPTOMS

BO3X ▸ Feel and sense very deep breathing. Sense the energy streaming and feel the spontaneous emotional releases that are following.

BO1X ▸ Hear and feel how repeated screaming provokes the same emotional release.

BO3X ▸ Sense and live a deep massage in spastic areas. Experience your pain with voice and facial expressions and in your body.

CLOSE YOUR EYES AND BO3X ▸ Sense and feel again how powerful is this way that permits one pressure or a single muscle spasm to promote a spontaneous outburst.

BO3X ▸ Feel and know the repressed emotion being released. Recognize the specific memory of a forgotten trauma or event attached to this emotion.

Note: Practice the following exercise once daily in the AM for 21 days.

BO3X ▸ Imagine and sense you are working with facial expressions and make faces into the mirror. Sense and see what is happening when you are rolling your eyes around, wiggling the face and forehead in rhythmic movements, stretching the eyes and mouth wide open, expressing various emotions by eye contact with an authority, mentor, or someone you love or like.

....

WE ARE EMBODIED BEINGS:
BY ELAINE WALDMAN, A REICH STUDENT ▸
FOR OVERCOMING SEXUAL INHIBITIONS

BO3X ▸ See and feel your mindbody connection as an expression of your total self.

BO3X ▸ Sense that your body is at first your past and your present. Sense that your body is your personal and interpersonal experience. Sense that your body is your conscious and non-conscious attitudes. Sense that your body is your motions and emotions.

BO3X ► See how the presence of opposites is evidence of each aspect of the individual.

BO3X ► Sense and know how when this oppositional dimension is energized, it can make contact with its polar counterpart.

BO3X ► Sense and feel these polar counterparts and know how when you find them, you move toward a new integration of your life force and a higher level of energy.

BO3X ► See yourself as a one-sided individual and sense how you tend to exhaust yourself in the struggle and become run down energetically.

BO3X ► Feel and know that we function at the same time on an integrated organismic level and as a single cell however complicated we experience ourselves to be.

BO3X ► Sense how the presence of organismic function is pulsation. Sense the expansion and contraction. Sense the charge and discharge. Sense the reaching out and pulling back. Sense the giving and the taking.

BO3X ► Sense and feel how our movements are regulated by the goals of pleasure and grounding.

BO3X ► Sense and know how we function only if there is a balance between charge and discharge.

BO3X ► Sense how our cells and our organs can act interdependently and when they do we are in perfect balance. When we are in perfect balance, our organs and cells are pulsating rhythmically.

BO3X ► Feel and sense how breathing in is charging up our energy level, and self-expression is discharging it.

BO1X ► Sense how the two are going simultaneously and how the amount of charge shows how much we are giving out.

BO1X ► Sense and know how we are in balance only when there is a charge and discharge.

BO3X ► See how the difference between health and illness is the difference in our pulsating processes.

BO3X ► Sense how the harmony between excitation and inhibition, as a functional unity, gives balance and grace to our lives.

BO3X ► See and know how death is the complete loss of such rhythmic excitation.

BO3X ► Sense how the mobility of our organism is manifested by the movement of the body fluids.

BO1X ► See and sense the movement of your blood.

BO1X ► See and sense the movement of your lymphatic fluids.

BO1X ► See and sense the movement of your intracellular fluids [fluids within cells].

BO1X ► See and sense the movement of your intercellular fluids [fluids between cells].

BO3X ► Feel and know how experiencing excitation is taking us beyond our anatomical boundaries into the midst of others' reaction with the world.

BO3X ► Feel and know how at the same time, we can become aware of the identity of ourselves with the world.

Power of Nothing
or Empire of Nothingness

*"I am not myself, but a lot of little selves. By possession
and passion, they tied me down. If we cut the links,
like a white bird, the Soul flies."*
-Colette, "Cerf Volant"

SEEING LIFE THROUGH A CRYSTAL EYE

BO3X ▸ Imagine that you are a hermit in a cave in the Himalayas. You have a crystal egg inside a reliquary*. You are hearing sounds of this egg. The sounds are grace and memory. You close the reliquary and hear from the mountains below robbers intending to come to the cave to steal the egg and murder you.

BO1X ▸ You leave the cave with the reliquary and see yourself escaping from the robbers by becoming a desert in the Himalayas. The robbers run right over you as they go into the cave. You then turn into a yak who passes near them. They see you and realize they have been tricked. As they come after you, you turn into a pack of Himalayan wolves.

BO1X ▸ Now see yourself as an eloping pair of lovers who are making their way to Varanasi [Holy City of India on the Ganges].

BO3X ▸ See yourself as an avenging monk on the road of truth. You first become a Zen monk who is sitting in zazen and under the stick of his teacher. You then become a Taoist monk developing your chi. See yourself developing all the powers that chi gives and in turn giving that to others. See yourself becoming very old, dying sweetly and returning to live again exactly the same life. Then become a Tantric monk having to fight the demons. Fight the first, then the second demon that are projections you have to vanquish. After vanquishing each, throw them into the abyss. Fight the third demon and see how many more there are and say how many more. Know that after vanquishing each, you have taken one step on your road. After the last demon, you are entering into the clear light. After absorbing the clear light, you find enlightenment and continue your pilgrimage.

BO3X ▸ You are the old monk traveling with the crystal egg. You are in Varanasi at the Kumbh Mela* and join the pilgrims washing in the Ganges at dawn. There are thousands of them. Above you is the stone staircase the pilgrims ascend between dawn and sunrise to celebrate the sunrise. Feel what they experience at the top of the staircase.

BO3X ▸ Far above the stone staircase is a high mountain. At the top of it sits a Buddha. In one leap, you jump up to the Buddha. You pluck out one of his eyes and sit in the hollow socket. Far below, you are the ascending pilgrims and their bodies floating in the Ganges. You become the eye of the Buddha and see how to deal with the robbers, whose intentions you must avenge. See how to arrange the wedding of the two lovers so their families in Varanasi are accepting and reconciling their marriage. Then see far in the distance, what is best for you now.

BO1X ▸ Jump down from the eye of the Buddha and replace the eye. As the old monk, with the crystal eye, make your way back to your Himalayan cave and return right where you began.

EYES THAT SEE EVERYWHERE FOR PROTECTION & KNOWING: FROM ALEXANDRA DAVID-NEEL*

BO3X ▸ See the Egyptian all-knowing eye Udjat* outside yourself. Reaching out into your right hand, delicately take the eye and slowly bring it to your forehead, placing it between your eyebrows. Look everywhere with this eye and see someone you wish to know. See laser light going from this eye and penetrating into the other, so you are able to know them perfectly in mind and body. Find out what you need to know. After, take the eye from your forehead delicately with both hands and sense its presence there. Stretch your hands way out in front of you, turn your hands over, and deposit the eye where it came from.

EYES OF THE ADVERSARY TO KNOW THE ANTAGONIST: FROM ALEXANDRA DAVID-NEEL

BO3X ▸ See your adversary before you. See that your entire body contains eyes, in every pore of your skin there is an eye. These eyes are protecting you. With these eyes you see directly into your adversary to know the power and plan of their behavior. Your eyes are not judging eyes, but knowing eyes. They are full of light, knowing what is in the adversary's mind. You plan your argument in advance of their knowing what they are going to say or do. It is important for you only to know your adversary's plan, not important to subdue or defeat the adversary. Do not feel angry or vengeful, but only need to counteract what might come from your adversary.

CLIFF OF SERENITY TO CLEAR DISTURBING EMOTIONS: FROM ALEXANDRA DAVID-NEEL

BO3X ▸ Find yourself at the base of a cliff at a beach. Know how you have gotten to the base. Afterward, look at the white cliff and with a sharp stone engrave the negative feelings that have been plaguing and bothering you. Engrave these traits deeply into the stone. Lay out a white sail on the beach beneath the cliff. Throw stones at the cliff where you have engraved your negative traits to break them up. Use a hammer and chisel to continue the job. See the stones breaking up and falling from the cliff into the white sail. Gather up the sail and tie the corners to make a bag.

Gather wood from shipwrecks at the bottom of the sea and make a boat. Load the bag of stones onto the boat and set off. Go through the waterways, meeting people of the different countries and relating to them by adopting a response that is different from the habitual traits in the bag. Eventually, turn into the Pacific Ocean. Go to its deepest part and drop the bag into the ocean, seeing it disappear from view. Feeling lighter, take the boat in the opposite direction through the Pacific back through waterways, stopping along the way to learn more about the people and to understand them. Arrive at the shore from where you started, then look at the fresh cliff and do not touch its freshness. Jump to the top of the cliff with your new lightness and there, in a meadow, let yourself be quiet and relaxed.

TÊTE-A-TÊTE, HEAD-TO-HEAD: REPAIRING FAMILY DISCORD

BO3X ▸ See and hear the core body part of your identity say something to the core body part of another person you know. Have the core part of this person say something to your core part. Imagine your core answering. What is the dialogue?

BO1X ▸ See yourself staring at the naked back of your father. Tell yourself what you see, feel, and do. Stay a long moment.

BO1X ▸ Now have your father staring at your naked back. What do you feel and do in this reversing of positions?

BO1X ▸ See yourself staring at the naked back of your mother. Now have your mother staring at your naked back. What is this reversing of positions telling you?

BO3X ▸ Imagine entering the body of your father or mother and traveling in to find their heart. What happens?

BO3X ▸ Imagine each parent entering your body. What happens when they find your heart?

BO3X ▸ Imagine what your head is saying to your father or mother's head.

BO3X ▸ Imagine what your heart is saying to your father or mother's heart.

BO3X ▸ Imagine what each part of your body is saying to each part of your parents' bodies.

EXERCISE FOR COUPLES:
USING BODY LANGUAGE FOR MARITAL ACCORD

Note: Each person does the exercise.

BO3X - Have the core of yourself speak to the core of your partner.

BO1X ▸ Have yourself enter the body of your partner. Find out what part of your body is irritating the other, and is turing him/her off. Ask the other what repair needs to be made.

BO1X ▸ Have your partner enter your body. Find out what part of his/her body is irritating you, and is turing you off. Tell the other what repair needs to be made.

BO1X ▸ Enter the body of your partner, and find the other's heart. Have his/her heart speak to your heart. Hear your heart's response and his/her response to you. Be aware of the dialogue.

HEART-TO-HEART:
REPAIRING FAMILY RELATIONSHIPS

BO2X ► What does your head say to your heart? What does your head say to another part of your body?

BO3X ► What does your head say to one of your parents' hearts?

BO1X ► What does your heart say to one of your parents' heads?

BO3X ► Imagine what any part of your mother says to your head. Imagine what any part of your father says to your head.

BO2X ► Know what your gut is saying to your mother or father.

BO2X ► Know what your gut is saying to any other part of your mother's or father's bodies.

BO3X ► Have a heart-to-heart conversation with a significant person. Hear the conversation and what each heart is saying to the other.

BO4X ► Imagine you are taking a shower with your mother and afterward with your father. Note what body parts are seen and what are avoided.

BO2X ► Imagine you are lying in bed between your mother and father. Pay attention to all you are sensing and feeling.

BO3X ► Into a mirror, see all the images of head-to-head and heart-to-heart that have touched you. See your attitude in front of you and make a correction.

BO3X ► Be in front of the mirror and live in the mirror your core experience of tête-a-tête and heart-to-heart, knowing how your behavior is connected with the images.

Personality

"With a twinkle in the eye I send a glance to the Absolute."
-Colette, "With a Twinkle"

HUMAN VARIABILITY

BO3X ► See a box filled with masks. Choose a mask and hold it in front of your face, but not touching your face. This is your persona. Say a word through the mask, then say your name through it. What sound does your name make?

BO3X ► See what it is like to wear a different mask for different people.

BO3X ► Having a mask in your hand, but not in front of your face, see the different masks you have to wear with other people.

BO1X ► See different people in front of you and having a mask in front of your face, having the choice of keeping or changing the mask. See what is the pattern of behavior you perform and what it is you want to express.

BO3X ► See, know, and live how the self is lived or experienced through the persona.

BO3X ► See and recognize the different parts of the self in mind, emotions, and body for what they are. Look at how they are arranged and how they are put together.

BO3X ► Look at your different parts in what is the mind, emotions, and body and see how they are placed in life and put together right now in life, in the world, in history, and in the universe.

BO1X ► See and know how the physical aspect of your constitution is set up and structured.

BO2X ▸ Know how these different parts are making an individual and know how being an individual is to be undivided. Feel yourself to be indivisible after this.

FEMALE PSYCHOLOGY

Note: Do these two exercises only once a year. Write down your responses and review them a year later.

BO3X ▸ Make a vase with clay. Take a stylus and imprint on the turning vase all you want to change in yourself in one year. Break the vase and throw its parts into the sea.

BO1X ▸ Make a vase and draw on it the symbols of what you'd like to change in yourself. Put the vase in an oven. When it is hard, break it and bury the broken pieces.

BO3X ▸ Into the mirror, see your self-portrait as superwoman.

BO1X ▸ Into the mirror, see your self-portrait as the American Indian, White Buffalo Woman*, living in harmony with the full circle of life.

BO1X ▸ Into the mirror, see your self-portrait as the Tibetan goddess Durga,* giving you power and justice.

BO1X ▸ Into the mirror, see your self-portrait as a woman heroine and know what in you is giving you results.

SUN AND SHADOW

BO3X ▸ Into the mirror, construct a model of sun and shadow.

BO1X ▸ Into the mirror, see yourself having the masculine qualities of assertiveness, dominance, competitiveness, and loudness.

BO1X ▸ Into the mirror, see yourself with the feminine qualities of openness and vulnerability, caring, and cooperation.

IMPOSED ON FROM THE OUTSIDE

BO3X ► See and feel yourself being an integrated psychological totality.

BO3X ► Look at Apollo, the sun god. See and know why he remains the prototype of lucid, enlightened wisdom.

CHARACTER: ACQUIRED TRAITS

Note: Character is the tool we use to inscribe our own traits and is not reflective of outside forces, which is persona or personality.

BO1X ► Know why we have to look at a prototype to recognize the given properties of body and consciousness.

BO3X ► Look at a tile and have a tool in your hand to engrave letters.

BO1X ► Have the tool engraving letters and see yourself engraving in you what you choose to engrave. See yourself now impressing what you like onto the world. Know what aspect of you is the self that puts this stamp on the world.

TEMPERAMENT: INBORN TRAITS

BO3X ► Looking into the mirror, see your character and personality traits. Temper these parts to obtain what you want of yourself and what is pleasing to you. Try to find the well-defined proportions and blend them. Know how incorrect or immoderate proportions result in ill-tempered behavior, which leads to bad humor or mood, which leads to mental disease.

BO3X ► Enter into the mirror to see the difference between men and women in style;

BO1X ► In degree of consciousness;

BO1X ► In emphasis;

BO1X ► In proportion and in the order of priority given to things.

ISIS*, GODDESS OF WISDOM

BO4X ▸ Feel and see yourself as the Goddess Isis, reassembling the dismembered body of Osiris*. See yourself as Isis, re-membering him.

BO3X ▸ Feel and know how remembrance is putting the different parts in at the right place and at the right time, to make them a living whole.

BO1X ▸ See, know, and feel how remembering is a restorative and creative act.

BO3X ▸ Know and feel how by remembering a love, you create the new, for you are bringing the forgotten one back to a new wholeness and by reinstalling him in the external world, you are bringing him into existence.

BO1X ▸ Feel and know how by immersing himself into the depths of a deep woman, man comes to know himself.

BO3X ▸ See and feel how by looking into the image of the deep consciousness, we come to know ourselves.

BO3X BREATHING OUT GREY SMOKE AND BREATHING IN BLUE LIGHT IN EACH CYCLE. Feel and know how a real woman is the vessel of transformation and transposition and why men who are seekers and runners-after-truth at first have to find the right woman.

Tree of Life

"Through the Tree of Life, the Vital force,
By the medium of Light is channeled."
-Colette, "Shaddai"

THE TREE OF LIFE:
FOR NEUROLOGICAL DISORDERS

BO3X ▸ Imagine a tree and see it as a synthesis of air, earth, water, and light. Sense the tree as dynamic life as opposed to the static or apparently static life of a stone.

BO3X ▸ See and feel the tree as being the world image.

BO3X ▸ See the tree forming the three worlds* and making communication between them possible.

BO1X ▸ See the tree giving access to solar power.

BO3X ▸ See, feel, and sense how the tree is rooted at the center of the earth and is in contact with inside waters.

BO3X ▸ Look at the growing of the tree in the world of time having rings. See how the branches show differentiation as they try to expand.

BO3X ▸ See an evergreen tree and know it is the image of everlasting. Look at a deciduous tree and know how it is an image of renewal and regeneration.

BO3X ▸ Sense how the unity and regenerative quality of the Tree of Life in the center of the Garden of Eden is opposed to but complementary of the deciduous Tree of Knowledge, with its teaching of good and evil.

BO3X ▸ See the Tree of Life and the Tree of Knowledge inverted upon one another, the Tree of Life upside down. See the Tree of Life with its roots spread as rays of sun in the air catching all cosmic energies and bringing them to the Tree of Knowledge, which directs them to the earth.

BO3X ► See and sense the reflection of these two worlds in one another. Sense their two natures but unique essence.

BO3X ► Sense how reversing of the Tree of Life is the way of illumination. Sense in this way, how the Tree of Life is the Tree of Light.

BO3X ► Sense the dew on the branches and leaves of your own tree and hear the voice of the dew.

BO3X ► See how the serpent around your tree is showing you your difficulties when trying to reach wisdom.

BO3X ► See that the serpent is tempting you to obtain knowledge, but is telling you how you may have it only if you are constantly changing your skin and regenerating.

BO3X ► Know that you cannot keep this knowledge only for yourself. See yourself taking a golden apple on the tree and parting it into as many pieces as there are people with whom you want to share your knowledge. Give every one of them their part of knowledge.

....

COME TO YOUR LIGHT

BO3X ►Sense and see that you are a crystal crossed by light. Describe your form, the rays coming to you and the rays going out of you.

BO3X ► As a crystal, hear the different sounds when different rays are touching you.

TO BECOME A TRANSPARENT CRYSTAL PALACE

BO3X ► Hear the glory of light hiding The Word.

BO1X ► Hear the voice telling This Word.

BO1X ► See that the meaning of your word is truth.

FROM EZEKIEL

BO3X ► See the light that is creating the four legs of the throne of truth.

BO1X ► See the light that is creating the four angels on each of the four legs.

BO1X ► See the light that is creating the four faces on each of the four angels.

BO1X ► See altogether the 64 faces of light.

BO3X ► See the 64 directions of space as arms of the world, sending light, peace, and health in every direction.

ARMS OF THE WORLD

BO3X ► Sense the victory and splendor that the arms of the world are ready to send, if you ask for them.

PILLAR OF CLOUDS

BO3X ► See the pillar of clouds concealing a mystery from you, and sense it behind you. See and sense the separation made by the husks of evil. Sense this separation as guarding the path of enlightenment.

THE NAME

BO3X ▸ See how your name is in you and in you is your name to give life and light to your study and enlivened life. See yourself studying to have your master fly in the sky.

LIGHT SHADOW

BO3X ▸ Sense in your light shadow, your principle of individuation and your garment. What is the difference?

BO3X ▸ Feel and know how this is your spiritual configuration and unique essence.

BO3X ▸ Sense and feel how the light shadow is a projection of your inside and the repository of the years you have to live.

BO3X ▸ Sense that it is as a garment for your soul, and is coming from your good deeds.

BO3X ▸ Feel, sense, and see your light shadow as your true self.

BO3X ▸ Sense and feel how this light shadow is permitting your three souls to work in you (your animal soul, higher self, and Spirit soul).

BO3X ▸ Know that without the protective light shadow, the soul may burn the body with its fierce radiance. Thank your light shadow for its protection.

BO3X ▸ Look at all your souls that have been initially woven into the curtain hanging before the Throne of Glory. What is the material of the curtain? Greet and welcome the souls, the living and the others.

BO3X ▸ Find your own soul woven and embroidered onto the curtain. See all its development since the first beginning from your past history to your future destiny.

BO3X ▸ Finding your own soul, see if it is revealing what you want to be. If not, look at one possible change and learn how to do it without hurting your soul or the old curtain.

BO3X ▸ Sense your responsibility to be the one to repair what has been woven since the beginning of time. Do it only if you feel you have to do it.

BO3X ▸ Look at all the souls, past, present and future. Look at all the souls of all your children and heirs. Follow every one in his or her life, now and into the near future.

FOREST OF FORGIVENESS

BO3X ▸ See yourself standing in front of a forest. See all who have hurt you coming out of the forest one at a time. Look each one in the eye and tell each of them how they have hurt you. Forgive each and see them disappear or forgive them and send them on their way.

FROM ONE MIND TO ANOTHER

BO3X ▸ See how love is a primal value for contact with others. See the others at first as an observer and see how it changes with love.

Search for Identity

*"…Choose a color for every day. Create in joy and purity
and stay happy."*

-Colette, "The Light of Lights"

TOO MUCH, TOO LITTLE

BO5X ▸ COUNTING SILENTLY FROM 5 TO 1, EACH OUT-BREATH BEING A
NEW NUMBER. See the number one as a lighthouse focusing light. Go to a circular mirror and see it as a lighthouse focusing light in and around you.

BO3X ▸ COUNTING SILENTLY FROM 3 TO 1, EACH OUT-BREATH BEING A
NEW NUMBER. Seeing a lighthouse in the mirror, focus the light on the personal
qualities you wish to change or burn away, using the light as a laser. Turn the mirror over and see the light focusing on those senses you wish to energize — your
senses of touching, hearing, smelling, tasting, seeing.

BO3X ▸ To experience each sense, use the light to focus all around you,
enhancing the specific sense or senses you want energized. (You can increase or
decrease each sense as you wish.)

BO3X ▸ COUNTING SILENTLY FROM 3 TO 1, EACH OUT-BREATH BEING A
NEW NUMBER. At 1, see yourself in the mirror becoming the lighthouse. See
there, positive emotion as a color; see there negative emotion as a color. Then see
the nuances of the negative-emotion color and use the lighthouse as a laser to
burn it away. Turn the mirror over and experience an emotion color you wish to
experience more deeply and see all the nuances of color your lighthouse opens up.

....

YOUR GUARDIAN ANGEL, WISE ADVISOR

BO3X ▸ See yourself going backwards into a mirror. See your shadow going
farther and farther away until it becomes a point. See the point disappearing.

BO1X ▸ See the point reappearing. Reconstruct your shadow and see it coming
out of the mirror, reuniting with you. See your Guardian Angel. Go through the day
with your Guardian Angel and thank it.

BO1X ► Push your Guardian Angel away violently or fragment it and see the pieces of shells. See if there is anything inside the shells.

BO1X ► See if you are keeping anything from before. See yourself as you are now.

BO3X ► See and know how we are the uniqueness of a moment of cosmic truth.

BO3X ► See and live the struggle that shows the agony of nature that makes us feel and recognize the way to cure the struggle.

BO3X ► See how truth requires us to be young.

BO3X ► See, feel, and know if all along your life you have had some stable qualities like being gregarious and assertive or if all along your life you have had the qualities of being introverted and anxious or if you have had the constant quality of being impulsive.

BO1X ► Feel and know if these constant traits are inherited, biological dispositions, influences from early childhood, or patterns of social roles or expectations.

BO1X ► See and know which traits you are locked into.

Introspection

"Infinite in space and time, we are free to find in everyone,
the perfect image to contemplate."
-Colette, "Prayer"

INNER JOURNEY

BO3X ▸ Live and know how the little self or ego-fulfillment is asking for immediate gratification.

BO1X ▸ Live how this self-fulfillment is a desire to get and not to give.

BO3X ▸ Live and know how self-fulfillment makes for a restless searching and spending.

BO3X ▸ Know and live how ego-fulfillment is asking for freedom, but is pushing us to avoid a lifestyle, commitments, and involvements, which would bring such freedom.

BO3X ▸ Feel and know how, when going to extremes, we become self-absorbed and are oriented and preoccupied only with the self (ego).

BO3X ▸ Feel and know the difference, when involved with the self, between a true search for self and self-indulgence that brings social alienation.

BO3X ▸ Feel and know the difference between introspecting and engaging in a search for awareness and meaning.

BO3X ▸ Recognize how when cutting with a previous form of life you like, you may feel empty or even bad.

BO3X ▸ See and know how working with images is a way of organizing reality and finding inside meaning.

BO3X ▸ Sense in yourself the battle of nature. Sense it as an agony of parts of yourself.

BO1X ▸ Recognize the way to repair and cure it.

BO3X ▸ Feel and know how you often seek what you call your problems because you need their gifts.

BREAKING WITH THE PAST

1. BO3X ▸ See yourself going backwards over a bridge, saying goodbye to those you have befriended, ignoring those who have used you, and forgiving those who have harmed you. When reaching the end of the bridge, throw a bomb that blows up the bridge between you and the past, the now and then. After doing this, turn and find a new direction and a new place for yourself in life.

2. BO3X ▸ Imagine the Hands of God taking away envy. Imagine the Hands of God taking away hatred. Imagine the Hands of God taking away rivalry. Imagine the Hands of God taking away regret. Imagine the Hands of God taking away guilt. Imagine the Hands of God taking away anxiety.

3. BO3X ▸ Imagine the Hands of God opening the doors to healing. Imagine the Hands of God opening the doors to tranquility. Imagine the Hands of God opening the doors to clarity. Imagine the Hands of God opening the doors to forgiveness. Imagine the Hands of God opening the doors to happiness. Imagine the Hands of God opening the doors to concrete material well-being. Imagine the Hands of God opening the doors to good fortune. Now the doors have been opened.

BO1X ▸ and imagine the Hands of God taking you by your shoulders and raising you up a thousand feet.

4. BO3X ▸ Take a star in your hands and put it in your heart. See and know the truth inside your heart.

Note: The above four exercises can be used specifically for dealing with depression.

5. BO3X ▸ Know what has made you the person you are now.

BO1X ▸ What are the two most important events in your life? Allow the images that are coming reveal you to yourself.

6. BO3X ▸ Recognize and live some place in your house. Recognize and live some event in your life. Recognize and live being with someone you know. Recognize and live some regret or remorse you cannot get rid of.

BO3X ▸ With a lasso, tie each of them separately.

BO1X ▸ Now tie all the lassoed images together. Open the lasso to free just that one still in your mind by tying it to something now happening. Then throw the lasso away, behind you.

7. BO3X ▸ See and know how to fulfill your possibilities. At this moment, you may change your self-esteem by any way that comes to you. Then you may change your sense of control over your life. Choose now the ultimate value that is now to guide your life.

8. BO3X ▸ If we are to totally give up our personal identification, experience how part of ourselves is always afraid of being swallowed up in the tide of wider consciousness.

9. BO3X ▸ See and live the childish fears and resentments brought into focus.

BO1X ▸ Sense them pushing us to show our distress so someone will have to protect us.

BO1X ▸ Live and recognize how by doing that, you have made yourself unhappy and dissatisfied.

10. BO3X ▸ See and feel how in knowing our imperfections, we create standards impossible to reach.

BO1X ▸ Sense how we feel that if we do not succeed at being the best, we are the complete opposite.

BO1X ▸ See that we often have focused on small issues to avoid the wider field.

BO3X ► Live how you are discovering the three different modes of insight:

1. focus on bringing inarticulate feelings into words;

2. focus on the way to easily focus your attention;

3. focus on a non-assertive will by psychic surrender.

BO3X ► Imagine how the function of will is to want not to push.

BO1X ► Live how this kind of will enables you to move from a narrow to a wide focus.

BO1X ► Live how this wider attention is coming from attending to something and yet wanting nothing from it.

BO3X ► Live and find your different mode of escaping attention in a positive way.

BO3X ► Focus on bodywork or art. Live how you perform brilliantly by putting your controlling mind out of the way.

BO3X ► Count your blessings and see yourself at the end of the day writing down in your journal the moments that have brought you happiness.

BO3X ► Count your blessings and see and feel yourself examining and reliving the delights of the day in your private life, work life, and outside contacts.

BO3X ► Feel and live that by examining possible happiness, you have found reasons for burdens, anxieties, fears, a sense of inadequacy, and constricted consciousness.

BO3X ► Live and know how you are discovering blind thinking and subliminal childish emotions, ideas, and patterns. See and know how by finding this blind thinking you reach clarity, expanded consciousness, and moments of transcendence.

BO3X ► See and live how by observing your inside and then your outside and through trial and sometimes by error, you are coming to some insights.

RESTORATION

BO3X ▸ Looking in a mirror, see what and who you are and recognize if your identity is based on an attachment to someone, some ideal, or some thing. IF THIS IS THE CASE, THEN:

BO3X ▸ Feel what happens when the cord is cut. See and feel how attachment makes you afraid of not being liked or of being left and that friendship is in part, hanging on.

BO1X ▸ Live how without fear of loss, all is available for friendship or union.

BO3X ▸ Picture one of your prize possessions, something you hold dear. Imagine it stolen or lost and picture the exact moment when you discover it gone. Notice your feelings, thoughts, and emotions.

BO3X ▸ Choose a minor annoyance that is bothering you physically.

BO1X ▸ What is the pattern that emerges when you are bothered or frustrated?

BO1X ▸ Now discover the root of this annoyance.

BO3X ▸ Live some period of suffering caused by attachment to a life situation.

BO1X ▸ Live some period of suffering caused by attachment, such as an athlete losing physical strength.

BO1X ▸ Live some period of suffering caused by attachment, such as a student facing graduation.

BO1X ▸ Live some period of suffering caused by attachment, such as a mother when her children are growing up.

BO1X ▸ Live some period of suffering caused by attachment, such as an unsuccessful writer.

BO1X ▸ Live these changes as partial emotional deaths.

BO1X ▸ Restore yourself from the loss by rebirthing or activating something you like to do better than anything else.

BO3X ▸ Imagine the first time you did this. Feel in your body all the related sensations.

BO1X ▸ Imagine mind-induced trouble or suffering. Image how rich your life will be without attachment to these feelings.

BO1X ▸ Now feel and live your mind-induced health.

BO1X ▸ Know how your state of health reflects your state of mind.

BO3X ▸ Into a mirror look at your body and notice places that are not in perfect order. Reconnect your state of mind with each of these black spots. What happens?

....

FROM *AS A MAN THINKETH:* BY JAMES ALLEN*

BO3X ▸ Sense and know the meaning of the phrase, "They, themselves, are makers of themselves."

BO1X ▸ Sense and know the meaning of the paraphrase, "You, yourself, are the maker of yourself."

BO3X ▸ See, feel, and know how the mind is the master weaver of the inner garment of character and of the outer garment of circumstance.

BO3X ▸ Become aware of the hidden seeds of thought.

BO3X ▸ See and sense how they spring forth into acts.

BO3X ▸ See, know, and feel how the act is the blossom of the thought and know how joy and suffering are its fruits.

BO3X ▸ See and know how that Godlike character is the natural result of your continued effort in "right thinking."

BO1X ▸ Know how in the armory of thought, you forge the weapons by which you destroy yourself.

BO1X ▸ Now, in the armory of thought, fashion the tools to build the heavenly mansions of joy, peace, and strength.

BO3X ► Know and see how you are the master of thought, the molder of character, and the maker and shaper of conditions, environment, and of your future destiny.

BO3X ► See how circumstances reveal you to yourself. See how you attract to yourself what you are, not what you want.

BO3X ► See your thoughts becoming the jailers imprisoning you.

BO1X ► See your thoughts becoming the angels of freedom liberating you.

BO3X ► See and know how the hidden soil-and-seeds of your being give birth to your circumstances.

BO1X ► Having realized this power, become the rightful master of yourself.

BO3X ► See, sense, feel, and live yourself harmonizing wish, prayer, thoughts, and actions.

BO3X ► Sense and know how the sole and supreme use of suffering is to purify, to burn out all that is useless and impure.

BO1X ► See how suffering is a result of mental disharmony.

BO1X ► Hear the sounds of harmony rising up from your heart to your throat and utter its sound.

BO3X ► See and recognize failure as a starting point or pathway to attainment.

BO1X ► See yourself attempting fearlessly, accomplishing masterfully, and thinking strongly.

BO1X ► Now mentally mark out a straight path to your purpose. Look neither right nor left and reach it.

NIMIR* AND THE WELL OF WISDOM: TO CREATE A NEW FUTURE

BO3X ► Imagine and see an enormous Nordic giant, called Nimir, guarding the Well of Wisdom. Ask him for permission to plunge into this special well to find old memories that bring you actual wisdom. When he agrees, thank him.

BO1X ► Throw yourself into the well like a missile, touching all valuable memories for an instant and omitting from your life those that do not serve your life. Do not compromise.

BO1X ► Look at each significant memory, which is bringing you knowledge about yourself. Take the memories with you as you ascend from the bottom of the well and return with the messages of the past. Bring the messages into the light, for your mission of today is to be clear and accomplished. When you have cleaned up all you have found, know this makes you mindful.

BO1X ► When leaving the well, make a promise to Nimir that you have not changed the level of the water, and also that you will seek a new home without attachments to those of the past, which have been useless.

TIME: WHY LIGHT IS CALLED DAY, DARKNESS CALLED NIGHT

BO3X ► See, know, and live how time is determined by its content.

BO1X ► Know why light is called day.

BO1X ► Know why darkness is called night.

Wisdom of The Body

"Now, my left and right, top and bottom, feel connected."
-Colette, "Essence of Reality"

HEALING BY BREATHING

BO3X ▸ Know and see how by making yourself conscious of your breathing, you permit yourself to get rid of hindering influences and to feel liberated.

BO3X ▸ Sense and know the subliminal feelings that are delivered.

BO3X ▸ Feel and know how by breathing out you are allowing sense perceptions to come out and be free.

BO3X ▸ See and feel how you don't have to correct the breathing pattern all at once, but you can use it as a starting point, even if it is a faulty one.

BO1X ▸ See and feel the inner movement of your natural breathing until the breath left to you returns to a normal pattern. Stay with this a long moment.

BO3X ▸ Sense the intimate connection of this breathing with your two nervous systems, the voluntary, consciously directed one and the involuntary, reactive one, which works without your mind.

BO1X ▸ Sense, feel, and know how the breath forms a bridge between the voluntary and involuntary nervous systems.

BO3X ▸ Know how by watching your breath you may learn to observe a normally involuntary function at work.

BO3X ▸ Know how by watching your breath, you learn how to exclude interferences and to help your self-regulating processes, such as yawning before becoming over-tired and sighing before becoming over-restricted.

BO3X ▸ Sense and know how our breathing pattern is expressing our inner situation. Know now what that situation is.

BO3X ▸ Sense and feel we are breathing irregularly when concentrating and focusing our attention. Know this is normal.

BO3X ▸ Feel and sense an emotional state. Be aware and see how your breathing is changing.

BO1X ▸ Sense and feel how your breathing is agitated in anger.

BO1X ▸ Sense and feel what is happening with an emotion of fear.

BO1X ▸ Feel and see how when feeling sad our breathing becomes choking or suffocating.

BO3X ▸ Sense how we are sighing when we are relieved. Sense now your breath becoming normal. Sense and feel how when at peace you are breathing with your diaphragm.

BO2X ▸ Sense how when in stress or maximum effort you are breathing with the chest.

BO1X ▸ Sense and feel how if we are not opening the chest cage we become anxious, inhibited, self-conscious and with a sense of inferiority.

BO3X ▸ Sense and know how when there is almost no exhalation, the abdomen is pulled in tightly.

BO1X ▸ See it like a bottle filled with consumed air. Open the bottle and breathe out in a safe and slow way. Be aware of your feelings.

BO2X ▸ See and sense how when abdominal breathing is disturbed, the inner life is disturbed.

BO3X ▸ Sense and know how the slow exhalation is reversing the habitual neurotic process.

BODY MOVEMENTS: FOR HEALING PARALYSIS

BO3X ▶ By breathing up and down your body you become aware of it. Focus your attention on your breathing. Feel how the air flows into your nose and mouth and down your throat. Feel your chest and belly expand as they receive this life-giving air. Image now that you are breathing into other parts of your body. Imagine the air flowing through your pelvis, then expanding in your belly and going down to your legs, your feet, and your toes, as they expand and contract a little. Now breathe into your shoulders, your arms, and your fingers. Notice how you feel.

CENTERING: BREATHING

BO3X ▶ Then breathe into your lower abdomen below your belly button, into the center from where all your movements are flowing. Now move slowly outward from the center. Be aware of how you move and feel when moving toward your center, then away from your center.

BO1X ▶ Now exaggerate and move slowly toward your inner then outer world.

BO1X ▶ Imagine yourself standing in a circle with a group of people. See yourself compressing into a tight ball, then expanding toward the world. Look toward a person in the group or toward a personal goal. See, feel, and sense yourself opening up to this person or goal and reaching it. Imagine yourself closing your eyes and opening them again toward another person or goal. Be aware of what goes on in this silent interaction. How do you feel? How are you and others moving and what do these movements express?

BO1X ▶ AND OPEN YOUR EYES.

NOW PHYSICALLY, STAND UP, AND BE AWARE THAT YOU ARE STANDING. EXPLORE THE TENSION YOU FEEL. REMAIN STANDING AND CLOSE YOUR EYES.

BO3X ▶ INTO THE TENSION AND RELEASE IT. Focus attention on your feet and legs and their contact with the ground. Be aware without moving how your weight is distributed between your feet. Is there more weight on the inside or outside edge? Notice any difference you feel between your feet. How do your feet contact the ground? Do your feet receive it, grip it, draw back from it? Now be aware of how your legs feel and notice any difference between them. How do they support your upper body and connect with your feet?

BO1X ▶ AND OPEN YOUR EYES AND SIT DOWN.

Knowing Ourselves Through Seeking and Returning

"Being in need of Realization,
To be saved I separate from those I love."
-Colette, "Springing Above"

BO3X ▸ Feel and know how to be a seeker is a blessing.

BO3X ▸ See and know how seeking is humanity's chance to grow.

BO3X ▸ Recognize and know why the seeker is the one who looks for more, the one with an active question.

BO3X ▸ See and feel why the seeker with a quest or a question is the hero.

BO1X ▸ See and know how the quest is not about seeking the unknown, but about seeking something we have not lost or forgotten.

BO3X ▸ Hear and know how this "Lost Chord" is still resounding in us.

BO1X ▸ Hear and feel how it affirms the wholeness of our identity.

BO1X ▸ Hear, see, and know why and how the restoration of our wholeness is possible.

BO3X ▸ Feel, know, and see how unity is the destiny of man.

BO3X ▸ Live the homeward journey of the Prodigal Son.

BO3X ▸ Know and live how returning is the basic human longing to see Paradise as our last home.

BO1X ▸ Recognize why the Garden of Eden is so far away in time and space and opposite to our human daily realities.

BO3X ▸ Know and live how the quest for transforming your destiny is the reunion of you with yourself.

BO1X ▸ Know how it is such a trial, that most of the traditions have put it in another world, in another life, which is on the other shore.

BO3X ▸ See and live how we have been created: He-us.

BO1X ▸ Know how being incomplete and unfinished is to be imperfect.

BO1X ▸ Know why it has been possible for Christians to name this incompleteness sin.

BO3X ▸ See why St. Augustine has named this incompleteness blessed, knowing how this imperfection is the possibility of becoming.

BO3X ▸ Live the possible potential given by the unfinished.

BO2X ▸ Now see yourself caught between the rocks of your own contradiction.

BO1X ▸ Now see how to pass through this contradiction and its incompleteness.

BO1X ▸ See yourself climbing up the branches of the Tree of Life. What do you see, feel, and know, when returning to this origin?

BO3X ▸ See yourself climbing up the rungs of the ladder on the staircase that reaches the heavens. In this process of transformation, pay attention to all the changes that may happen.

BO3X ▸ See yourself crossing a maze. Someone you trust has given you a ball of thread, which you attach to the tree at the entrance. When you reach the center, know if you want to return or not return.

BO3X ▸ See yourself walking on the Rainbow Bridge. Know that all you see has to be remembered. Feel how the Rainbow Bridge is so fragile that the guides are hardening it with their breath. Know, feel, and see how transformed you are.

BO3X ▸ See yourself as Lancelot. See how you are walking at the edge of a sword blade to reach where the Lady is held captive.

BO1X ▸ See yourself as the Bodhidarma* crossing the Ocean of Transmigration*. How is this crossing made?

BO3X ▸ See the bridge projected from the highest peak of judgment at the center of the world. See how at its entrance, the soul is awaited by an angel who is its true, fulfilled identity.

BO3X ▸ See some hideous creature there, trying to stop the soul and your soul has to vanquish it. Remember that the hero is victorious and alone.

EXILE FROM INDIA

BO3X ▸ See yourself crossing the abyss, which is only an arrow shot across. You must know what is the arrow and how it is to be released.

EXILE FROM AFRICA

BO3X ▸ See yourself crossing a large torrent by creating a bridge made from a chain of arrows, which you shoot alternately to the near and far shores.

EXILE FROM NATIVE AMERICA

BO3X ▸ Looking at this created ladder, ask yourself what is the nature of such arrows.

EXILE FROM JAPAN

BO3X ▸ See the Japanese master of archery instructing his greatest pupil, you, to shoot down a star. When this is done, pay attention to your feelings. Now hear the master of archery directing you to do the same thing without using an arrow or a bow.

CROSSINGS

BO3X ▸ Feel and know how you are crossing the bridge at another kind of speed that is possible only when you forget the self. Know how the bridge is within and is crossed by taking risks.

BO3X ▸ See yourself at the seashore jumping onto a ray of a moonbeam from wave to wave.

BO3X ▸ Know and experience what has been told in the ancient traditions that "He who would be chief, let him be the bridge."

BO3X ▸ See how when crossed, the bridge must disappear for him who crossed it. Now see yourself as the Buddha told it, "Forget the raft when the other shore is gained."

BO1X ▸ Know how at the instant we reach our inside, we have to forget our outside and the way in which we reached the inside.

BO3X ▸ Feel and know how the bridge exists only in the moment between what was and what will be.

BO3X ▸ See how once crossed, the bridge is no longer needed because both shores in ourselves are joined.

BO3X ► See and know how by traveling, at last you come to the source of the river.

BO1X ► Feel how the separation has disappeared and how as the hero, you now become whole.

BO3X ► Know how you have not left one world for the other, but found how one is part of the other.

BO3X ► Feel and know how by crossing the bridge, you have liberated yourself, becoming free of all dimensions and all limitations.

THE HEAVENLY POLE

BO3X ► See yourself traveling in a dark forest having lost the north.

BO1X ► Live yourself going out of the forest and living the two-fold twilight.

BO3X ► Looking at this virtual, or potential existence, find the Heavenly Pole.

BO1X ► See, find, and live the Midnight Sun. See, find, and live the Night of Light, "the black light," the lucid earth, "the luminous blackness," the dark noontide.

BO3X ► Live and feel the Night of the Super Being, Unknowable of the Origin of Origins, the Light filled with a sense of Divinity.

BO3X ► Live the start of bi-unity with the Heavenly Partner in the concrete, spiritual universe of the heavenly earth.

BO3X ► Know how the soul lives in the twilight beacon.

BO3X ► Feel and know how by climbing, the peak is being drawn toward the center by touching the straight path.

BO3X ► Live how the distress of the twilight is the refusal of the hostile dawn.

BO1X ► Live and know how this distress is an expression of the powerlessness of the man who is no longer oriented to the Heavenly Pole.

BO3X ► See how you enter the Cloud of Unknowing* that gives birth to light.

THE RETURN

BO3X ► See yourself as the man of light, as the bi-unity, who is the guided and the guide.

BO3X ► Know and live "The Power That Is In Thee" in each one of us.

BO3X ► See and know the One whose name is Perfect Nature, as the Philosophic Angel, your Initiator and Tutor.

Life Within Life

"Eternity joins me when I join the Eternal Soul.
But, how to live eternity, now, and fulfill the duties
assigned by the will of the Eternal?"
-Colette, "Eternity"

BO3X ▸ Live in yourself the Freudian stages as a road that is: oral, anal, phallic, and genital.

BO2X ▸ Follow this inside road in reverse, staying in each of these places for the purpose of feeling and finding a source of energy.

BO3X ▸ Know that they are no longer in the past, but activated in the present time and are alive.

BO3X ▸ See and sense the muscles of your face contracting and notice how the eyes, ears, and nostrils are opening. How does it affect your face and the rest of your body?

BO3X ▸ See how you are manipulating to avoid being manipulated.

BO3X ▸ See yourself play-acting in front of people who have importance in your life.

BO1X ▸ Feel and know how your true self is suffocating when cut from any meaningful social intercourse.

BO2X ▸ Sense how the environment becomes more and more unreal as you have distanced yourself from the events of your life.

BO3X ▸ Know how when this process accelerates, the self creates a further split. Then a gulf is created and sometimes an abyss is felt.

BO3X ▸ Feel how we are haunted by our own play-acting and by our flight from trying to become what we truly are or would be.

BO3X ▸ See how when the guilt mounts, we silence the inside voice by distraction, alcohol, walking around, or doing a lot of little things to avoid facing reality.

BO3X ▸ See how when the effect of the manipulation ceases, we are left alone with the emptiness of ourselves.

BO3X ▸ Feel how the inner self retreats from interaction when the self is split.

BO3X ▸ See yourself leaving your body, now perceived as empty, false, or dead.

COLETTE'S DEVELOPMENT

BO2X ▸ See yourself dealing with the other in a way that is pure theater, while the inner self looks on as a scientific observer.

BO2X ▸ Know how the perception is then unreal and the action is futile.

BO3X ▸ See yourself retreating into fantasy at work or in love. See how you establish a false self that performs the necessary movements to succeed at your tasks.

BO1X ▸ Know and see yourself at age three or four, engaged in this process. Recognize how it is to go on further in your life, if not stopped. See it now, then, and in the future.

SPLITS IN THE PSYCHE: FROM R. D. LAING*

BO2X ▸ Sense and live the moment when your psyche split.

BO2X ▸ See the false selves created by the psyche in an attempt to protect itself.

BO2X ▸ See and live the manipulations that are provoking the psyche to protect itself.

BO3X ▸ See and know yourself and others in direct interaction.

BO1X ► Feel you and they engaging each other in an immediate way.

BO1X ► Sense and know how the perception is real.

BO1X ► Recognize then how your action is meaningful.

BO1X ► Feel how you, yourself, are embodied and vital.

BO1X ► See and recognize how this direct interaction is almost never taking place.

BO1X ► See and feel that we are whole for almost no one, least of all for ourselves.

BO1X ► See and live the world of social roles, interactions, rituals, and elaborate games played in the way you are living.

BO2X ► See and live how you are forced to protect yourself by creating a false-self system.

BO3X ► Repair any or all of these as needed by any means you imaginally discover.

....

PREPARATION FOR OVERCOMING DEATH

BO3X ► Going from linear duration to vertical eternity.

BO1X ► See and live the fears, doubts, regrets, and guilts that have pushed you to emptiness and loneliness.

BO3X ► See and live how these fears are fears of the unknown and fears of death.

BO1X ► See, feel, and know that to fight against these fears, we have to go out of the linear time of every-day life by living intensely in the present.

BO3X ► Know that by living such an intense present moment, you live life as a vertical eternity.

BO3X ► See, feel, and know that to live this intense present in a vertical eternity, we have to change the way we are now living our inner life.

BO3X ▸ See yourself constructing a vertical line from earth to heaven, instant by instant. See each instant as a point.

BO1X ▸ See and feel how in living one point after another point, you are in a fully lived life.

BO3X ▸ Feel and sense at each point of the vertical lived life that you are newly born again in the eternity of the moment.

···

DEFEATING DEATH:
FROM GABRIEL GARCIA MARQUEZ*

BO3X ▸ Imagine you have taken an eternal ticket for a train that never arrives at its destination.

BO3X ▸ See how the position of sitting with crossed legs is bringing you directly to death by forms of mortification that never stop.

BO3X ▸ See how you have been born with the attraction to desire and love. Sense it.

BO3X ▸ See and feel some concentrated idea of love.

BO1X ▸ Sense and know how love is the human way to fight and shield against death.

BO3X ▸ See and feel how to resist the past you have to live in the present.

BO3X ▸ Sense in yourself the lives of your ancestors and decide to accept from them only what is yours.

BO3X ▸ See yourself deciphering the manuscript of the future beginning with the instant you are now living.

BO3X ▸ Feel and know how this moment is your moment. Know how it is eternal and cannot be repeated.

BO1X ▸ See, sense, and feel that the light of now is the only possession you have, and the only certainty.

BO3X ▸ Sense how valued events of the past are coexisting with the present in the same instant. See how the light of the past is the same as the light of now.

BO3X ▸ By seeing it, consider how stress is your individual reaction to conditions that disturb and disrupt your natural equilibrium. See this stress as worry, anxiety, and rebellion that reflect themselves in biological dysfunction.

....

LIFE AND LIGHT

BO1X ▸ See yourself becoming moderate and obtaining balance in all dimensions of living, except when searching for truth.

BO1X ▸ See yourself setting aside a half-minute, twice a day, for quieting Imagery.

BO1X ▸ See yourself reducing now the frequency of stressful life changes.

BO3X ▸ See how you accept your physical and emotional limitations for the ability to improve.

BO3X ▸ See and feel how you break the stress spiral by balancing work and play and being less serious.

BO1X ▸ See how you have fun when you are light-hearted.

BO3X ▸ See yourself taking perspective when an intense or painful scene is happening.

BO3X ▸ See how when in a stressful situation you are using Imagery or a healthy outlet like walking, gardening, slowly drinking a glass of water, slowly washing your hands.

BO3X ► See how you are using the same healthy outlets in conflict, emotional tension, or frustration. See yourself smiling a true smile.

BO3X ► Sense how the muscles of a true smile are really working.

BO3X ► Sense, feel, and know that life is your first teacher and your medium for self-expression by means of change and growth.

BO1X ► Live how seriousness is making you heavy, while images are making you light and alive.

LIGHT WITH IMAGES

BO3X ► See images as vibrations. Hear their clear language bringing order to your body. By the imagery process, see how you can create or maintain the condition of the body in either good or poor health.

BO1X ► See and live how the decision is yours, nearly always, consciously.

BO3X ► See how you decide to accept the large responsibility for what is your state of health or lifestyle or for any needy arrangement.

BO3X ► See how you agree to move gradually into the direction of change.

BO3X ► See and know with clear images if you are taking stimulants or doing stimulation exercises to mask a conflict or trouble. If so, see this conflict and know what to do for some unfulfilled need.

BO3X ► See and know with clear images if you are taking depressants or suppressing yourself. Find the reason and see yourself getting rid of it in your own way.

DEATH TO LIFE: NATURAL ENDING
BY CROSSING THE BRIDGE

BO3X ▸ Disengagement: See yourself withdrawing from one customary life routine.

BO3X ▸ Disidentification: Live the loss of your accepted definition of who he and she is. See them with new eyes.

BO3X ▸ Disenchantment: Live the discovery that someone or something you are dependent upon is not as you thought and is now insufficient.

BO3X ▸ Disorientation: Feel and see yourself at a moment when in losing all sense of what to do, you lose your actual self-image and where to go next.

....

LIGHT ▸ THE WONDER OF LIFE

BO3X ▸ Feel, sense, and know that you have a body.

BO3X ▸ Sense how you are this body among other bodies.

BO3X ▸ See, sense, and live your anatomical and physiological body.

BO3X ▸ See and live how you are feeling your body and all of your being for themselves.

BO3X ▸ Live and recognize your own joy as the scintillating sign that you are on your way and how this way is the right one.

BO3X ► Feel this joy as the vibration of the body, the heart, and the mind that are bringing you up to Spirit.

BO1X ► Sense that this joy is of the same quality as that of the naive one, of a young child or of the fullness of true lovers.

BO3X ► Feel and see this joy as the promise of life and know how this eternal joy is only of the instant.

BO1X ► Feel and know how this instant of joy is the marvel of life, which is bringing us above ourselves.

BO3X ► Feel and know how discovering the hidden marvel of this instant of joy is the reason for all forms of quest.

BO3X ► Sense, feel, and know how everything valuable begins with the body to allow what is valuable to jump out of the body.

WHAT TO DO TO REACH SPIRIT

BO3X ► Sense and recognize how we are seeking moderation to try to find more acceptable outside ways.

BO1X ► Feel how we do not have to go outside of ourselves to find new ways of enjoyment and truth.

BO3X ► See and know how all asceticism is built on the initial joy coming from the body.

BO1X ► Feel and know how by stopping this joy, we find a higher level of joy which is permitting the leap to Spirit.

BO3X ► Live and know how feeling your body specifically for itself is happening only by living by the inside.

BO1X ► Know and live how more of being comes when the emptiness that is pushing you outside is filled.

BO3X ▸ Know and live how by believing the manmade world to be the source of our internal melody, we lose our personal reality and power.

BO1X ▸ The Remedy: Live, sense, and know how by living the body from the outside, you store memories and block emotions. See yourself changing that.

FROM ONE MIND TO ANOTHER

BO3X ▸ See how love is a primal value to have contact with others. See at first the other as an observer and see how it changes with love.

LES VOYAGES: BY JULES ROMAINS* ▸ MEETING THE MINDS THROUGH LOVE

BO3X ▸ See yourself giving in to the direction of the one you love. See them sensing your love. STOP and recognize yourself.

BO1X ▸ See and sense their love melding with your love.

BO3X ▸ Imaginally contact someone you love. IF POSSIBLE, ASK THAT PERSON IN WAKING LIKE, IF THEY FELT THE CONTACT.

BO3X ▸ Discover an image permitting a supernatural contact.

BO1X ▸ Feel and know how prayer is the way to experience this transcendental contact. Say a short prayer.

BO3X ▸ Imagine you are drawing a white circle. See it as a space of light.

BO1X ▸ Enter the circle of light and wait for the Divine Light. Sense the Divine Light as a flow of life descending on you and into you. Say a short, silent prayer.

BO1X ▸ Go out of the circle of light. Erase it and let the crystal clear rain wash this place.

BO3X ▸ Sense how you and the one you love are of one mind. Send this one connected mind to other connected minds. Send all the minds you have met to the only One Mind.

Living in The Moment

"In this state of balance, for one moment I reach the unity."
-Colette, "Essence of Reality"

JOY: THE HIDDEN MARVEL

BO3X ► Live and recognize your own purpose in life and for now, your own joy, as the scintillating sign that you are on your way and that this way is the right one.

BO3X ► Feel this joy as the vibration of the body, the heart, and the mind that are bringing you up to Spirit.

BO3X ► Feel and know how this instant of joy is the marvel of life, bringing us above ourselves. Feel and know how discovering the hidden marvel of the instant of joy is the reason for all forms of quest.

BO3X ► Feel and see this joy as the promise of life. Know how this eternal joy is only of the instant.

BO3X ► Imagine yourself lying down, getting in touch with how your body feels.

BO3X ► Know, feel, and sense how everything valuable is beginning in the body and is jumping out of the body.

BO3X ► Feel and recognize how we are going out from the natural way to find more acceptable outside ways.

BO3X ► Feel and know how we do not have to go out to find new ways of enjoyment. We can find enjoyment by recognizing the inside joy.

BO3X ► Feel and know how by stopping it, we reach a higher level of joy that is named Spirit.

REST IN IMMOBILITY:
IMPORTANCE OF POSTURE AS A HEALING AGENT

BO3X ► Feel and know how in meditation specific thoughts of time or the posture itself may be the only healing agents.

BO3X ► Find and see the best posture for healing some inside disorder. Feel and know how long to hold this posture to sense well-being in your body.

BO1X ► Give your body the order to remember this length of time. Do this posture two times more. See and feel the disorder disappear at the third time, when you hold this specific posture.

BO3X ► Sense in yourself the physiological effect of immobility. Feel and know how refraining from movement for a specific length of time is strengthening your will.

BO1X ► Feel, recognize, and know how the importance is not only in the length of time, but in the purpose and the direction of your intention.

BO3X ► Feel how this very short time of rest is the real elixir of life by its liberating effect when it reaches the center of pleasure in the brain.

BO3X ► Feel and know how richness is given in the immediacy of spontaneity.

BEAUTY AND MAGNIFICENCE: FOR WELL-BEING

BO3X ► See and know the beauty and magnificence that are in you. Keep this in mind and feel only images of health, strength, success, kindness, goodness, joy, love. Sense their abundance.

THE DUALITY OF UNCERTAINTY

BO3X ▸ See yourself at the same time a person of action and a person of thought.

BO1X ▸ See these two main sides of your nature.

BO3X ▸ Look at the two faces of Janus*, the one looking at the past and the one looking at the future.

BO1X ▸ Feel your ego while at the same time being your alter ego (second self; opposite side of the personality). What do you want to be?

BO3X ▸ See and feel being at the same time in life and without life. What do you do?

BO3X ▸ See the God Shu* of Egypt uniting you with yourself. See him giving you and the other you the two feathers of his headband and holding the sky in his hands, not letting it fall on you.

....

THE EMBRYO OF IMMORTALITY

BO3X ▸ See the energy from the hollow parts of your body. Sense and gather this energy. Envelop it with your hands. Now embrace this embryo with your arms.

BO1X ▸ See this vital energy concentrating and becoming only breathing.

BO1X ▸ Live the movement of the breathing until you are not feeling or sensing it.

BO3X ▸ Sense the disappearance of your breathing as it becomes transformed into spiritual power. Feel deeply this spiritual power in your own body.

BO3X ▸ Feel the spiritual power in yourself and do with it what you want. Keep it spiritual, if you wish, or use it for intellectual purposes or body power. Its use is in your hands. Feel deeply the power of its being in your hands. Breathe out totally and return to a perfect vacuity or emptiness.

BO1X ▸ Return now to perfect emptiness, feeling the breathing below the navel, above the navel, in the neck and the mouth.

BO3X ▸ Know if you have realized some higher knowledge here and now in this state of emptiness.

BO1X ▸ Know if you have gained purification of being by overcoming grief, sorrow, and lamentation; by destruction or suffering; and of having reached the right path.

THE PAST AND ETERNITY: FINDING THE MOMENT

BO3X ▸ See, sense, know and live how the only way to live the present is to stop living with the past. It is possible only if you pass from the horizontal plane of everyday life to the vertical life of Spirit. Take the present moment and lift it up to eternity seven times.

Exercises of the Spiritual Heart

*"Floating as a cloud, blue stars crossing me, I slide to this new
Point where, you and me joining, are free…"*
-Colette, "Jewel of the Night"

WASH AWAY AND BROOM

REPEAT THIS FIRST EXERCISE, ONCE IN THE MORNING, FOR SEVEN DAYS.

BO3X ▶ Wash away or broom some place in your house, someone you know who is disturbing you, some inside imbalance, some regret, some physical ache that you don't know how to get rid of, some event you cannot forget.

BO3X ▶ Hear and feel the voice of the Inside Observer, the Egyptian Ka*, as the Will Toward Light between your heart and solar plexus.

BO3X ▶ Feel, sense, and live the Inside Observer, as a presence that quiets and calms anxiety and takes away the painful sense of uncertainty, insecurity, impotence, rancor, resentment, and pessimism.

BO3X ▶ Feel and know how this Will Toward Light is at first to make peace, so you must clean out all in you that prevents communion.

BO3X ▶ Feel, sense, and know how this place in your body between the heart and the solar plexus is the tabernacle where you must quietly concentrate to recognize the Inside Presence in order to hear its voice and feel its vital warmth.

BO3X ▶ Feel and know how this feeling of the Presence is the Vital Force, helping us overcome obstacles, if we deeply focus upon it with careful attention.

BO3X ▶ Know how it is important for us to identify this Presence in our own Spiritual Heart as the Heart of the Universe, which is our Cosmic Source of Light and Life.

BO3X ▶ Feel and know how direct communion with this reality brings peace and how the peacemaker is the heart.

BO3X ▸ Know and feel how by having confidence in our heart, we allow it to make communion between opposite rhythms, avoiding discharge and discordance. Know and feel how this permits communion between opposites to have full effect.

BO3X ▸ Feel and know how only by concentrating on the place between the heart and the solar plexus do we overcome grievances or anxiety and make simple the complications of our daily life.

BO3X ▸ Know, feel, and see how when the heart has won this useful victory, it is on the way to Light.

QUEST FOR REALITY

BO3X ▸ See and feel how simplicity of the heart is detachment. See yourself letting all that is not essential fall away -- intellectual richness, prejudice, and beliefs.

BO3X ▸ Feel free to undertake the quest of reality with the open-heartedness of a child.

BO3X ▸ Know how these acts of renunciation have to be free and how nothing can be non-spontaneous on this Path of Light.

BO3X ▸ Know how only the limit of our desires makes the limit of our enrichment on the Path of Light.

BO3X ▸ Know and sense how only a transmutation is able to bring a solution to the eternal question of loneliness, sadness, old age, disease, and death.

BO3X ▸ Know and sense how transpersonal states happen only when we forget ourselves and our appearances, and by sweeping away fears and anxiety we break with an insufficient form of life.

BO3X ▸ Feel and know how seeing and living such a break doesn't make you break into pieces, but is a re-awakening that gives you power.

BO3X ▸ Feel and know this process of breaking by brooming away fear and anxiety, and accept the possible transmutation to bring immediate joy and peace.

Resurrection of The Body

"Pulled up by your prayer – I am lifted up to a space of absolute quietness. There I am returned to primeval unity."
-Colette, "Healing"

HOW TO SUMMON YOUR INNER ALLY

BO3X ▶ Imagine yourself climbing up a ladder one step at a time and as you do, on each step drop something disturbing or disagreeable, finding yourself feeling free of all that is not who you really are.

BO1X ▶ Imagine a large, clear, quiet space, knowing by all your senses the reality of this place. When you feel this place is yours, call for knowledge from one of the possible beings: human, animal, or plant, living in this space.

BO1X ▶ The one who is coming is your natural ally, your guide and adviser. If you don't see this form or if what you see is disagreeable, put it behind an impenetrable barrier and call for another guide.

BO3X ▶ Befriend your guide in the best way you know. Feed it, give it flowers, caress it, and ask its name to know if it is male or female. Remember, this image belongs to your own inner self and you are in charge of it. Ask the guide if it wants to meet you daily for a week. Ask the guide to demonstrate a sign of its power and then to release you from a difficulty, a malaise, or a thorny problem — or to give you the right answer to a question. Remember, you are talking to a part of you that has become unveiled.

BODY MOVEMENTS: TO RETARD AGING

BO3X ▶ Focus your attention on your body and letting go so your body can do whatever it wants to do without planning or direction. As you focus your attention on your body, become aware of parts that want to move.

BO1X ▶ Let this or these parts move in any way it or they want — gracefully, awkwardly, flowingly — anything that feels right for the parts you are moving. These moving parts may bring other parts into movement as well.

BO1X ▶ Some movements may change and develop into other movements before they stop. As some movements stop, others may emerge or your body may want to rest or pause for a while. Continue to focus your attention on your body and let it do what it wants.

BO3X ▸ Some sounds and images may occur. Let them become part of your movements. Let them emerge and see what develops. See how you limit and inhibit yourself and notice the parts of your body that are tense and held in. After imaging positions you like and dislike, see what happens when imaging them with music.

TOWARD & AWAY

BO3X ▸ Imagine something attracting you so much that you would like to move toward it. Visualize it clearly. Be aware of how you feel and how your body feels. Now let your feelings flow into your slow movements toward it. Pay attention to how your body moves and feels toward this thing that attracts you and stay touching it and contacting it in whichever way you want. Now move slowly away from this thing and let your movements show you if you are still attracted to it, even as you are moving away.

BO3X ▸ Now stay where you are and imagine that very close to you is something specific that repels you strongly — something you want to move away from. See it clearly, recognize all your feelings about this thing, and express what you are feeling through your face. Now let your feelings express that you are flying away from this thing, being aware of how you feel. Now move again toward and away from this thing that repels you, experiencing clearly your feelings. Be aware of how you feel and move as you approach this thing and discover what it is like. Discover what it is that repels you, then discover something you can appreciate — something that actually attracts you toward it — and discover more about this thing. Now moving slowly be aware of how you are moving and feeling.

TENSING

BO3X ▸ Imagine yourself lying down. Focus your attention on your body. Feel where your body feels comfortable and at ease and where does it feel less comfortable or ill at ease? Now for a few seconds, tense your body as hard as possible. Breathe out, letting go completely. Do this three times.

COCOON

BO3X ▸ Find yourself in a cocoon. Explore your existence inside the cocoon. Know what your cocoon is like and how you feel there. Know how much space you have and how you can move around inside it. Now break the cocoon and find your way out. Be aware of how you feel emerging into the world. Stretch in any way that seems comfortable. With each stretch, emit a sound. Now become the sound and let it flow back into your stretching. Feel all the different ways of stretching and sounding in your body.

GRAVITY

BO3X ▸ See yourself stretch out of your cocoon again, elongating and moving slowly out of gravity. See how this force is pulling you and transmitted through the body to whatever part is supporting you. Feel your whole body responding to the pull of gravity on your position. Now imagine the pull of gravity doubling, that you are very heavy and every movement is a considerable effort. Against this tremendous energy, pull yourself to standing position and then sink down again to rest on the ground. Now imagine that the pull of gravity is reduced to half normal. You are very light and your body is moving effortlessly.

EXPLORING MOVEMENT AND SOUND

BO3X ▸ Feel yourself allowing movement to flow into your body. Let each part of your body be moving in whatever way is compatible for you. Hear the sounds associated with each movement. Explore the movement and sound together in many ways: swaying, twisting, jerking, rocking, undulating, rotating, flowing. Go on moving in whatever way is comfortable. Now make whatever sound you feel like making inwardly and let the sound flow into your movement. Now imagine pairing up with someone for a short dialogue of sound and movement.

BO1X ▸ See yourself finding a new partner and interacting with her or him through sounds and movements. Be aware how your sounds and movements differ with this new partner.

EXPLORING MOVEMENT AND SOUND: DANCE

BO3X ▸ Sitting in a comfortable position, get in touch with your physical existence. Know that each breath has a purpose and direction. Notice what is going on in your body. Imagine you are alone at the edge of a large, clear, quiet, and calm meadow with the sun above you and all the space to dance. Look at your meadow. Be aware of your feelings and begin to dance freely. Now see in this space another dancer, dancing. He or she has seen you and is offering to show you how to dance. You are free to accept, share, or reject this dance. See how the two of you are dancing together in the green, clear, quiet, large meadow.

EXPLORING MOVEMENT AND SOUND: EVOLUTION

BO3X ▸ See yourself lying down. Imagine you are inert matter at the bottom of a pre-historic sea. Feel the currents of water. Hear the raging, rushing sea-waves. Feel the water flowing over your inert surface. Now, as life develops, see and feel yourself becoming a seaweed or underwater plant. Listen to the drumming of the water and let this sound flow through your body and into your movements as the water flows into you. Now become a simple animal that crawls along the bottom of the sea. Move slowly toward the land. Let the sound of the waves move you. Now you reach land and grow four legs. Hear the sound of the wind along with the drumming of the water. Begin to explore your existence and the way you are moving as a land animal. Now gradually become upright on two legs and explore the way you move and exist as a two-legged animal. Hear all the sounds around and continue to move and see how you interact with the other two-legged animals.

BO1X ▸ Become the lotus and the shaft of light.

BODY MOVEMENT: SEPARATION/CONNECTION

BO3X ► Explore your physical sensations and what is going on inside you. Begin reaching out with your hands and feet and exploring the space around you. Do you feel like staying alone or do you desire to explore further and connect with someone else? If you do, move around and touch someone's hand. If you feel a return touch, you may choose to stay in this contact as one organism. Move around and if you like, absorb others into this organism who choose to join. You may continue touching and remaining as one organism with one another and then separating until you are alone again. Experience again being yourself and alone.

BODY MOVEMENT: INCOMPLETION

BO3X ► Imagine yourself sitting with a group. Look at half the group standing and moving around as if they are incomplete. Hear the sounds in you and around you, when the group is moving.

BO3X ► Now see half the people who are sitting get up and complete one of the incomplete beings with his movements and actions until each incomplete being is completed by another incomplete being.

BO3X ► See and feel each incomplete being interacting with another complete being. Sense this interaction. Feel well.

DIALOGUE AND MOVEMENT

BO3X ► See yourself in a group. Pair up with someone. Be aware of how you feel and what is going on with this one, looking at or touching him or her. Now silently say goodbye to your partner through movement and go to another person, moving, speaking, and parting. Silently say goodbye.

BO1X ► Imagine you feel sad and you choose a partner who feels joy. Be aware of how each of you is expressing sadness and joy. Switch places so sadness becomes joy and joy becomes sadness. Now make the opposite feelings occur. Notice how you are both becoming well balanced.

BO1X ► Imagine you feel unemotional and choose a partner who feels emotional. Be aware of how each of you is expressing unemotional and emotional. Switch places so unemotional becomes emotional and emotional becomes unemotional. Now make the opposite feelings occur, creating balance within both of you.

BO1X ► Imagine you feel passive and choose a partner who feels active. Be aware of how each of you is expressing passive and active. Switch places so passive becomes active and active becomes passive. Now make the opposite feelings occur, creating balance within both of you.

BO1X ► Imagine you feel impatient and choose a partner who feels patient. Become aware of how each of you is expressing impatient and patient. Switch places so impatient becomes patient and patient becomes impatient. Now have the opposite feelings occur, creating balance within both of you.

BO1X ► Imagine you feel hating and choose a partner who feels loving. Be aware of how each of you is expressing hating and loving. Switch places, so hating becomes loving and loving becomes hating. Now have the opposite feelings occur, creating balance within both of you.

BO1X ► Imagine you feel upset and choose a partner who feels calm. Be aware of how each of you is expressing upset and calm. Switch places, so upset becomes calm and calm becomes upset. Now make the opposite feelings occur, creating balance within both of you.

BO1X ► Imagine you feel rejecting and choose a partner who feels accepting. Be aware of how each of you is expressing rejecting and accepting. Switch places, so rejecting becomes accepting and accepting becomes rejecting. Now have the opposite feelings occur, creating balance within both of you.

BO1X ► Imagine you feel non-spontaneous and choose a partner who feels spontaneous. Be aware of how each of you is expressing non-spontaneous and spontaneous. Switch places, so non-spontaneous becomes spontaneous and spontaneous becomes non- spontaneous. Now make the opposite feelings occur, creating balance within both of you.

BO1X ▸ Imagine you feel annoyed and choose a partner who feels excited. Be aware of how each of you is expressing annoyed and excited. Switch places, so annoyed becomes excited and excited becomes annoyed. Now have the opposite feelings occur, creating balance within both of you.

CAPTURING THE HEART:
FOR CARDIAC ARRHYTHMIA

BO3X ▸ Imagine your heart is running in front and before you. What are you feeling?

BO1X ▸ Imagine that you elongate your arms and catch your heart with your long hands. Sense it beating in your hands until you feel that its pace is even.

BO1X ▸ Return your heart into its place in your body very delicately and thank it for reintegrating into your chest easily.

BO3X ▸ See your head upright and turned around 180 degrees to face behind you. What are you hearing when listening to your heart? What are you hearing when listening with your eyes down? What are you hearing when listening with your eyes up?

BO1X ▸ When you have found the sensation of feelings well balanced, caress your heart and make it anew.

RENEWING THE HEART ▸ OPERATION:
FOR HEALING THE HEART

BO3X ▸ You are in front of a large white staircase. You climb up to the fifth step and stay there. Open your chest, delicately pick up your heart and hold it in your left hand.

BO1X ▸ With the tip of the fingers of your right hand, clean your heart of its spots or bruises and any irregularities or difficulties of function. Caress now the heart with your right hand. Sense the kindness and warmth of your right hand protecting the heart by the knowledge and wisdom of the hand. Know how the hand is teaching the heart to behave and to understand the way.

BO1X ► Slowly climb up five more steps. Looking at your heart, see that it is bright and strong.

BO1X ► Sense the weight of your heart. Delicately put your renewed heart in place and close your chest. Sense how your renewed heart makes you alive and lively. Look at yourself and see how you are. Slowly return down the steps. See and feel the changes in yourself.

TRAVEL OF THE ADULT HEART

BO3X ► See your heart under your left shoulder, under the skin on the bone. The bone is strengthened and filled with energy from the love of your mother. The heart rests on the left shoulder then it travels across the collarbone to the right shoulder. It stays there for a second and starts descending the staircase of your ribs, descending all twelve ribs. What is happening as it descends down each rib? Then it reaches the diaphragm. It travels along the diaphragm gently and lightly, reaching the solar plexus. From the solar plexus, it radiates to all the organs and the whole body, making the blood healthy and then the heart travels along the rest of the diaphragm to the left and up to its rightful place in the chest. It is radiant, red, and strong, like the best ruby.

LIKE WATER IN A CRYSTAL CUP

BO3X ► Imagine you are opening your chest and seeing your heart the way you like. Caress it delicately. See it becoming a good and healthy shape and a healthy color. Now see a crystal vase in the shape of the heart. Inside it is multi-colored water, like a running river. You hear its sound as you pour it on you from above your head, all along your face, along your body and all along the inside of your body through your open mouth. Feel well and renewed.

ARROW IN THE HEART

BO3X ► You have an arrow in your heart. What are you seeing, sensing, and feeling? Take the arrow out and send it into the eye of a cyclone. What is happening? What are you sensing, feeling, knowing? Then send your arrow out of the cyclone into the stratosphere.

LIBERATION OF THE HEART

BO3X ▸ You have a quiver holding arrows. With a bow and a flaming arrow, surround the one you want to listen to you and tell him or her all the most hidden feelings from your heart.

"FROM MY FLESH I WILL SEE GOD": FROM JOB

BO3X ▸ See the eye of your heart sending messages to the eyes of your skin. Feel, sense, and understand how or what is inside and outside.

"I AM GIVING YOU A NEW HEART AND A NEW SOUL": FROM EZEKIEL

BO3X ▸ Know the purpose of your new heart and new soul. Feel and sense that the heart is put into you by God. See how from this point, you can reach Spirit.

FROM *SPACE, TIME, AND MEDICINE:* BY LARRY DOSSEY*

BO3X ▸ Imagine and know that your body is not an object and cannot be localized in space.

BO3X ▸ Feel and know your body in dynamic relationship with the universe and with all other bodies.

BO1X ▸ Sense and feel this physical exchange.

BO3X ▸ See and feel yourself involved in the biological dance of life.

BO1X ▸ Feel and know how each particle can only be understood in relation to all the other particles.

SYMPTOMS

PLACE YOUR HANDS ON YOUR LAP.

BO3X ▸ See your hands and be aware of all the sensations coming from them. See them as electrodes.

BO2X ▸ Become your right hand. Know that you are your right hand.

BO1X ▸ Become your left hand. Know that you are your left hand. Now have your right hand say something to your left hand and your left hand say something to your right hand. Have the hands answer each other.

BO3X ▸ Feel the interdependence of the hands. Sense how they are cooperating. Feel the flow of energy going to the arms, shoulders, and neck. Feel if there is some tension between the hands.

BO2X ▸ Be aware of how the possible tension is returning back to you and is driving you to bad habits and to symptoms.

BO1X ▸ Be conscious of the role of the bad habits in your life.

BO1X ▸ Be aware of some physical symptom. Try to increase this symptom by focusing on it. Then eliminate the symptom by trying to: gradually feel the reduction of the symptom, letting go, forgetting, fighting, explaining the way it has to change. Feel the symptom reducing until it disappears. Be honest and open to the message this symptom is sending to you and others. Be honest about making the change this message is giving to you.

To Live: Self Healing

"Beyond the appearance, the hidden Truth calls me.
Beyond the seven skies, eternity here and now finds me."
-Colette, "Beyond"

BO3X COUNTING BACKWARDS FROM 3 TO 1, EACH OUT-BREATH BEING A NEW NUMBER. Look into a mirror. See how going backwards and upside-down is changing all the old habits and is cleansing you out.

BO3X ▸ See your bad feelings against others.

BO1X ▸ See yourself understanding these others. In doing so, know how the bad feelings began.

BO3X ▸ Feel and see your own anger as ugly and destroying.

BO3X ▸ See and feel yourself having the freedom and happiness that comes from stopping anger or changing it to something positive.

TO ALLOW GOD TO WORK THROUGH YOU BY CLEANSING YOU

BO3X ▸ See yourself with your own real beauty.

BO1X ▸ See how lying to yourself is destroying and distorting your real beauty.

BO1X ▸ See yourself cleansing out the lies and feelings that come from lying.

BO3X ▸ See all the impurities in yourself as impersonal and imperfect manifestations of the universal aspect of life.

BO3X ▸ Know and see all impurities as impersonal and imperfect manifestations of the universal aspect of life and know how they have come into you. See how you are suppressing them, if you do not transform them.

BO3X ▸ COUNTING BACKWARDS FROM 3 TO 1, EACH OUT-BREATH BEING A NEW NUMBER. Look at yourself in the mirror and see yourself touching each part of your body, beginning from your neck going downward, including all the extremities. See who is causing you a pain or burden and to whom you are a pain or burden. Remove that being from yourself, pushing him or her away to the left or in any direction that is comfortable for you.

BO3X ▸ See Adam and Eve in the Garden of Eden after God has withdrawn.

BO1X ▸ See yourself right now.

BO1X ▸ See your image in a mirror. Look at this image going backwards further and further from you. See it becoming a shadow.

BO1X ▸ Looking into the mirror, see the shadow and reconstruct it piece by piece, becoming your Guide, Guardian Angel, or Wise Advisor. Ask him or her for a piece of advice.

....

RABBI NACHMAN'S BRIDGE

BO3X ▸ See yourself as an old man about to cross a narrow bridge that is swaying from side-to-side as the river rushes below, engorged by a storm. Grasp the handrail and begin to cross. As you get to the center, a monster arises and tries to grab you. Then other monsters arise. As you move on, the devil stands before you on the bridge. You look him straight in the eye and walk over him. Then cross to the other side.

....

HEALING

BO3X ▸ Into a mirror look at evil and guilt. See yourself refusing to accept evil and guilt.

BO1X ▸ Clean out the mirror to the left with your left hand.

BO3X ▸ Turn over the mirror and see the goodness that is appearing in place of evil and guilt. Rest with this goodness, becoming assured of its eventual perfect accomplishment. See it done.

BO3X ► Look up and see yourself climbing a tall ladder to see behind the clouds. What do you see?

BO1X ► From behind the clouds, see what you feel guilty about.

BO1X ► Know that standard of guilt to which you respond.

BO3X ► See how by often making the world your apparent adversary, you have fought only yourself.

BO1X ► See your mistake. Know what you see.

BO3X ► See how the depth of your belief in injustice and tragedy may be the mark of ignorance.

BO3X ► See yourself not isolated, but a part of all.

BO1X ► Keep in mind only images of health, kindness, goodness, and love.

BO1X ► Sense and see their abundance.

BO3X ► Know and feel that what you accept is delivered to you by your all-knowing mind.

BO3X ► See, observe, and accept only what you decide is good for you and not harmful to others.

USING CONFLICT FOR HEALING

BO3X ► Know and feel how each partner in a conflict has the right to say, "I want to live this way. I am not content. I want to live this way."

BO3X ► See, hear, and feel yourself saying yes or no in a conflict.

BO3X ► Know how by feeling free to say yes or no, you are in a better position to negotiate differences.

BO3X ► Know how our intensity of feelings creates discomfort with the other's deferring values and behavior.

BO1X ▸ See yourself struggling through differences to go to an acceptable solution.

BO3X ▸ Know how our life is a puzzle and how we are learning the greatest truth about ourselves, when we recognize the pieces and put them in place.

BO3X ▸ Feel how by recognizing the placement of the pieces in our puzzle, we are:

BO1X ▸ expanding our frame of reference.

BO1X ▸ finding a vehicle for our evolution.

BO1X ▸ practicing this skill in an emotional and fearful contact that strengthens our ability to take risks in other areas of our lives.

BO3X ▸ Live and know how each little anger and disgust is an opportunity to see how we can liberate ourselves and our love from imposed self-constraints.

....

GROWTH

BO3X ▸ See yourself being threatened by the growth of your partner. See how this fear of change is understandable, but know that the fear is unrealistic.

BO3X ▸ Feel and know how our greatest chance for permanence lies in our ability to handle change.

BO3X ▸ Feel and recognize how we have to manage with these opposing or differing forces: the urge toward growth with risk taking, and the urge toward stability with stasis.

PRAYER: CREATING A SPACE FOR SILENCE

BO3X ▸ See, feel, and sense that the only praise worthy of God is silence.

BO3X ▸ Sense and feel how by tracing a white circle, you create a space.

BO1X ▸ See and feel how being in this space renews you.

BO1X ▸ In this space, have a short, silent prayer.

BO1X ▸ Be ready now to receive Divine Grace.

BO3X ▸ See and know that you receive Divine Grace when you feel a flow of life force.

BO3X ▸ When feeling this plentitude, know that the Divine Influx is passing through you in deep silence.

....

GIFT

BO3X ▸ See a rainbow coming from your lower abdomen, going to all the people you love. See a specific color going to the person you love, then walk to that person.

BO3X ▸ Tracing the Path of Light of the Rainbow with your feet and hands, paint a picture of what you want. Walk this Path of Light toward this desire.

A New Education

"The double message is coming to me, one of rigor, one of mercy."
-Colette, "Counter-Point"

CHANGES

BO3X ► Imagine it is morning and you are cleaning your bedroom, changing in it what you want to change. Begin by cleaning the ceiling and the walls. Now identify all that is no longer necessary for your purpose in life. Take it from the room and throw it away.

BO3X ► See before you a mirror and see yourself sending onto this mirror the clear number one.

BO1X ► And in the mirror look at your own light dimming your light and hiding your brightness.

BO3X ► See yourself clearly having repented all the wrongs you have done. Feel your heart now at rest.

BO1X ► Know that to keep this state of rest, you have never to return to the old errors or the old memories.

BO3X ► Feel and live why a great sage has said that in anger you have to remember love.

BO3X ► Recognize and live some disturbing images of a place in your house, and an event in your life.

BO1X ► See someone you know who is disturbing to you, then have some remorse. See some regret you cannot let go.

BO1X ► See places on your body where there is some physical pain.

BO1X ► With a lasso, confine each pain separately, then tie them up together.

BO1X ► Open the lasso and throw away the pain that has been the most disturbing and has created the lack of stillness in your mind. Become aware now of how your mind is behaving.

BO3X ► Imagine an object belonging to a different or unordinary world. Describe it.

BO1X ▸ Try to live degrees of change from something that is now important to you.

BO1X ▸ See and live yourself going from complete objectivity to subjectivity.

See how this is making you light, fresh, and bouncing.

BO3X ▸ Look at yourself having the intention to be full and whole like an egg.

BO3X ▸ See yourself as an iceboat cutting ice and being free. See yourself now in front of a wide, clear, quiet space.

BO3X ▸ See and sense yourself feeling badly because (1) you have had to cut from a habitual form of life or (2) you have had to cut from someone or something important to you or (3) you have had to cut from some house you have liked. Look at any one of these and imaginally join your hands on your heart and with your fingers capture the feelings that are attached to this other life and time…

BO1X …and throw it away, smiling at it, telling it "You belong to another life" and you have to be free to live this new life.

BO1X ▸ See yourself now sewing a beautiful patch at the place of your heart, replacing what you have taken away that was precious.

BO3X ▸ See, sense, and feel yourself climbing down the back staircase of a place you like or have lived in.

BO1X ▸ See yourself now going around to the front of the house, climbing up by the front staircase.

BO3X ▸ See and feel yourself looking at an aquarium. Keep these feelings for yourself.

ROMANTIC LOVE

BO3X ▸ Know and feel how romantic love is the pathway not only to emotional or sexual happiness, but also to the higher reaches of human growth.

BO3X ▸ See and live the changing form of intimate romantic relationship in the light of the growing interest of authenticity. See and live the changing form of intimate romantic relationship in the light of the growing interest of self-knowledge. See and live the changing form of intimate romantic relationship in the light of the growing interest of individual power. See and live the changing form of intimate romantic relationship in the light of the growing interest of paradox. See and live the changing form of intimate romantic relationship in the light of the growing interest of responsibility. See and live the changing form of intimate romantic relationship in the light of the growing interest of search for meaning.

BO3X ▸ Feel and know how in this period of cultural upheaval, we have to make peace with uncertainty.

BO1X ▸ See and know how to obtain this peace, we need to give up the attempt to control each other and give up the need to be right.

BO3X ▸ See and live how accepting uncertainty is an opportunity for personal transformation.

BO3X ▸ Feel and know how the root of romantic love is not sex but commitment.

BO3X ▸ Live how this commitment to and with a person is the golden path to growth and integrity.

BO3X ▸ See and know how romantic love is an ideal within our power to reach.

BO1X ▸ Live and feel how we reach it by effort of personal evolution and maturity.

BO3 ▸ See and live a fresh alternative in these contemporary issues: sexual choice, whether to marry, whether to have children, the conflict between love and work, age differences.

BO3X ▸ Know and live how loving someone is not a sufficient reason for making a commitment to a relationship with this person.

BO3X ▸ See, know, and feel the following reasons for romantic love: shared worldview, sense of life, having affinities, appropriate level of maturity, true self-esteem, and to feel lovable.

BO3X ▸ Live and feel how without self-respect, we cannot be worthy of happiness.

BO3X ▸ Live how the love affair with yourself is indisputable.

BO3X ▸ Feel, sense, and know how our inner image is our destiny and the blueprint of our future.

BO3X ▸ Know how maturity is necessary to recognize that our feelings are earned and do not come from something or someone outside yourself.

BO3X ▸ See and live how when relationship is good it makes us less likely to blame others for our changing feelings.

BO3X ▸ Live and know how disappointment comes from seeking security in relationships.

BO1X ▸ Live and know how disappointment comes from seeking relationship as the primary source of satisfaction.

BO3X ▸ Live and see how the value of relationship lies in gaining awareness.

BO1X ▸ See and know how by gaining awareness we become more real.

BO1X ▸ See and know how by gaining awareness we are not hiding one from the other.

BO1X ▸ See and know how by gaining awareness, we may resist attraction to become more real.

FROM MORTAL SADNESS TO DIVINE JOY

BO3X ▸ See yourself breathing out fear and growing cheerful.

BO3X ▸ See yourself choosing only one of these goods of the world: richness, possessions, money, security, comfort.

BO1X ▸ Know how making a living is not choosing life.

BO3X ▸ Live and know that the scientific fight for knowledge is habitually a fight for possession and power.

BO3X ▸ Live and know the difference between sincerity, reality, and evidence and recognize their relativity in everyday life.

BO1X ▸ Know the difference between all of this and truth.

BO3X ▸ See and feel how in our everyday life, being happy seems unusual.

BO1X ▸ See and live how behind a state of well-being is the feeling of guilt, that master of all other feelings that comes in to hide what we are living.

BO3X ▸ See and live for yourself the disturbance you experience by viewing television each day about disasters, horrors, exploitation of the weak, earthquakes, revolutions, and wars. Recognize your lack of power connected with your wish to help. Feel this inside tension.

BO3X ▸ See and live how our main activities are related to the need to forget and divert our mind and/or to be thoughtless.

BO3X ▸ Sense and know the difference between being over-excited, feeling lucky, and growing cheerful.

BO1X ▸ See and live how floundering in these states is connected with the appearance of a different state of mind.

BO3X ▸ Know as the Buddha and other sages have said how only a change is able to bring a solution to the eternal questions and problems of our lives: loneliness, sadness, old age, disease, and death.

BO3X ▸ Live and see these possible transpersonal states happening only when we forget ourselves and our appearances by breaking with a significant way of life and by crossing the bridge to the different and the unknown.

BO3X ▸ Feel and know how the seeing and living of such a break doesn't make us broken into pieces, but is uniting us by giving us power.

BO3X ▸ Feel and know how this process of breaking is accepting the possible change and is bringing immediate joy.

Identity and Self Identity

"The waterfall from High is thrown on you like a hurricane.
In the thunder, listen for the small voice."
-Colette, "The One Voice"

CONDITION OF THE PROPHETIC EXPERIENCE

BO3X ▸ See, sense, feel, live, and know yourself in perfect neurological and psychological condition.

BO3X ▸ See, live, and know your physical fortitude.

BO3X ▸ Among all your images, learn and know how to discriminate between hallucinations; fulfilling visions, and transcendental experiences, those called supernatural or beyond the ordinary.

BO3X ▸ Feel and know how to distinguish all desires from all ambitions. Recognize them for what they are.

BO3X ▸ Know and live as the prophet, how not to enter into a prophetic state when angry or violent.

BO1X ▸ Know and live as the prophet, how not to enter into the prophetic state when proud of being a person of vision.

BO1X ▸ Know and live as the prophet, how not to enter into the prophetic state when distracted.

BO1X ▸ Know and live as the prophet, how not to enter into the prophetic state when sad or mournful.

BO3X ▸ Live and know as the prophet, the truth that you are not performing voluntary miracles, but are waiting for the Will of God with a sign confirming His response to your request.

BO3X ▸ Feel as the prophet drawing down the Divine Grace and becoming an earth-dwelling messenger.

BO3X ▸ Know and sense that you are assuming this function only as part of the Divine Plan.

GAME OF GAMES: REVERSING THE VALUES

BO3X ▸ Feel and know how we control what we perceive.

BO1X ▸ See and live the difference between what we perceive and what actually exists, and the difference between what we perceive and what we actually do.

BHAGAVAD GITA

BO3X ▸ See how delusion arises from anger and fear. How do you repair it?

BO1X ▸ Feel, see, and live how loss of memory comes from delusion. Understand why.

BO3X ▸ See and know how the discriminative faculty is ruined from loss of memory.

BO3X ▸ See and know how the mind perishes from loss of the discriminative faculty.

TAO MEDITATION

BO3X ▸ See and feel how you will see clarity, if you close your eyes.

BO3X ▸ Sense and know how you will hear truth, if you cease to listen.

BO3X ► Feel and know how your heart will sing, if you are silent.

BO3X ► Feel and know how you will find union, if you seek no contact.

BO3X ► Feel and know how you will need no strength, if you are gentle.

BO3X ► Feel and know how you will achieve all things, if you are patient.

BO3X ► See and feel how you will remain entire, if you are humble.

THE BROKEN HEART:
BY RABBI MENACHEM MENDEL OF KOTZK*

"Nothing Is As Perfect As A Broken Heart"
-Rabbi Menachem Mendel

BO3X ► See yourself walking and as you go, hear the sound of your heart.

BO3X ► Know it is the sound of the best of you.

BO3X ► Sense the sound diminishing under a deep pain or grief.

BO3X ► Hear and recognize how the sound of your heart is more beautiful now.

RUNNING YOUR HEART OUT

BO3X ► See the star in your heart.

BO1X ► Hear its little palpitation.

BO1X ► Recognize how it is sounding as your Inner Voice.

BO1X ► See and sense the malaise of everyday life disappearing by this awareness.

BO3X ► See the star in your heart.

BO1X ► Imagine you are hearing and seeing your fright becoming light.

GALAXY

BO3X ► Imagine your heart amongst the stars, receiving the stellar light that draws the energy from all the other galaxies. Sense and feel your heart becoming rejuvenated, refreshed, and strong. See your heart back in your chest. Sense and feel what happens.

MOTION AND EMOTION

BO3X ► See and live how without emotion there is no motion.

BO3X ► See and feel your anger becoming the motion for whatever you want to realize.

BO3X ► Feel and know how rage and despair are the forces moving the world.

BO3X ► See and know how the regeneration of the world comes from these forces.

BO3X ► See and feel yourself in a small sailboat under a storm and notice what you are doing to get out of it without great damage.

BO3X ► See and know how if human beings are a large part of the problems causing the catastrophes of the planet, then human beings are the answer.

BO1X ► Sense how you may be one of these beings.

BO3X ► See yourself looking at flying, soaring, rising water that is more beautiful than any human being may be.

BO1X ► Sense how under the sun you are more transparent and crystalline than this flying water.

BO1X ► Sense how the poets or the artists are the ones most able to fix this one instant of beauty and magnificence.

BO3X ► Feel and know we are separate from each other even if we want to be united to each other.

BO1X ► Feel how love is the only cohesive element.

Quest for Hidden Meaning

"If I dive, I reach the Spirit of Delight.
At the surface I am bounced with beams of Light."
-Colette, "Fountain of Wisdom"

LOST JEWEL

BO3X ► Imagine how to return a dear one or your prince or princess to life, you have to find the only and unique precious stone hidden somewhere in the infinite world. What do you do? Where do you find it? How to you feel? What is happening?

LOST WORD

BO3X ► Imagine how in your quest for meaning you discover a book hidden somewhere long ago. Where do you find it? What is the title of the book? What is the word you have to find to learn what you need to know? What does it tell you? Know how this word has been forgotten or lost.

JAR OF AMBROSIA

BO3X ► Imagine you are traveling along the Greek Islands looking for the jar of ambrosia hidden and preserved for you since thousands of years ago. Where are you finding it? How are you opening it now to taste the ambrosia? Know what is happening to you after you have smelled and tasted the primordial ambrosia.

LOST GARDEN

BO3X ► You are walking your road back to the garden. See the entrance guarded by the angel with the flaming, turning sword. Try to pass through the fire and note what stays at the threshold. How to you feel?

BO1X ▸ Look directly at this gate and ask its name. Pass slowly through this gate and feel and know what you are leaving behind by this passage and what you are learning by this passage.

BO1X ▸ Know what you want to find hidden in the garden. Know and feel the primordial perfection here in this enclosed space.

BO1X ▸ Know what qualities you have had to develop to pass your way back to this center and what trials you have surpassed.

BO1X ▸ Feel and know how by regaining the garden you return to unity.

LOST LOVE

BO3X ▸ See yourself as the White Knight wandering around the world to find the princess raped by the Black Knight.

BO1X ▸ See how you have to fight the dragon.

BO1X ▸ See yourself crossing the abyss on the edge of a sword.

BO1X ▸ See yourself vanquishing the guardian of the tower.

BO1X ▸ See yourself watching the beautiful princess and bringing her back to her family circle.

GRAIL: FOR OVERCOMING DEPRESSION

BO3X ▸ Feel yourself as a young knight mounted on a horse. Feel and know how your spirit is guiding your body.

BO3X ▸ Feel and know that your quest is the journey of your soul.

BO3X ▸ See and live your travel in this world of temptation, obstacles, and trials. Know how they are building your character.

BO3X ▸ Feel yourself as the savior with miraculous powers to fight against evil.

BO3X ▸ Feel and know the sadness and the loneliness of being different.

BO3X ▸ Know how abandoning and being alone are the price to pay for the return to primordial unity.

BO3X ▸ See and know that whatever you conquer, you must leave it behind to go onward. See and know that you must always accept that separation follows union or reunion because you always must return to the world and change it.

....

SYNAGOGUE OF TOLEDO: FOR ANY SKIN DISORDER

BO3X ▸ See yourself at the door of the Synagogue of Toledo. You are surprised to see very aged, ugly, wrinkled old men who are sick and poor. Many of their eyes are full of anger. They are dressed in dirty clothes. They enter the synagogue and there on the floor are entwined circles of light under their feet and on the walls.

BO1X ▸ You enter the synagogue and stay near the back wall. In the center, you see a double red ladder.

BO1X ▸ See the men ascending and as they do, see them transforming into young men without wrinkles, having glowing skin and becoming radiant. As they reach the top of the ladder, they fly upwards toward the ceiling, where they see words inscribed.

BO1X ▸ See them now descending, maintaining all their changes. You leave the synagogue and watch them exit, keeping all the changes for them and for yourself.

Alone With the One: By Colette ▶ Union With God

"My self cast away, space is made for God...
He is ever present to me as to every one..."
-Colette, "Unbounded"

INVISIBILITY

BO3X ▶ Imagine a crystal in your hands. Make it grow to the size of a door and enter it. Imagine a metallic object in your hands. Make it grow to the size of a door.

OPEN YOUR EYES and see the image of a person in the room. Merge with them. Look above and below to gather all possible energies. See a spot on the wall or ceiling and watch clouds form around it. Draw a cloud around you and spin as you disappear and the cloud becomes a neutral color.

CLOSE YOUR EYES, looking into a mirror, see a spinning cloud.

MY TWIN

BO3X ▶ Feel and sense being intoxicated by God.

BO1X ▶ Know God is looking at you from far away.

BO3X ▶ See, live, and know God is bringing from the beyond, the way to step into eternity.

BI-REALITY

BO1X ▶ Become united, then live in two places at the same time: with family, children, friends, events, moments.

BO1X ▶ Then live where multiplicity finishes, where everybody and everything are one.

BO3X ▶ In this central uniting, see that evil is only part of the whole.

BO1X ▶ In the central unity, see and feel how Cain is the brother of the good.

ETERNITY

BO3X ▸ See, sense, live, feel, and experience that to live eternity now is to fulfill the duties assigned by the Will of the Eternal.

THE ONLY ONE

BO3X ▸ Hear the call of the Only One. Hear the One and lose the One. Then sense the One in the transparent, empty space residing in vibrant, clear light and tranquil harmony.

BO3X ▸ Know and feel the love of family, children, and friends as precious gifts. Know that these relationships are the pure reflection of the Only True and Perfect.

BO1X ▸ Feel and know how beauty and joy are signs that in letting go, you have left behind what was the least to reach the best.

LOVE

BO3X ▸ See, sense, and live two loves living side-by-side. One is the model of the other or its image.

BO1X ▸ See how each love asks for all of you. See how to keep the balance, giving God what is God's, giving to your beloved what is due by right of birth.

BO1X ▸ But know that one day...

GENEALOGY

BO3X ▸ See and sense how I am my ancestors and descendants.

BO1X ▸ See and know how without this continuation, the universe ceases to exist.

BO1X ▸ Observe it and it is.

CANDLE

BO3X ▸ Know how if you cannot be a star in the heavens, you can be a candle burning in this cloudy valley.

BO1X ▸ See and know if you want God's light one day, extinguish this little candle, modestly glowing in the night.

GATHERING ROSES

BO3X ▸ Be in a jungle garden gathering roses in the colors of peach, apricot, and cherry. Sense the light, freshness, and radiance crowned by an aura of beauty and glory.

OPEN AND RE-CLOSE YOUR EYES

BO3X ▸ With these roses, do as the girls did in ancient days, making the wine wise men were drinking to recreate what is wrong in the world by rejecting evil.

OPEN AND RE-CLOSE YOUR EYES

BO3X ▸ See how the women dressed in this ancient garb are bringing grace downwards, the roses becoming stars.

EARTHQUAKE IN HIS MIND

BO3X ▸ You are the stormy wind.

BO1X ▸ You are the great white cloud.

BO1X ▸ You are the flashing fire.

BO1X ▸ You are the earthquake in God's mind.

OPEN AND RE-CLOSE YOUR EYES

BO3X ▸ He says that in your golden silk garment, you bring the full moon onto the earth.

OPEN AND RE-CLOSE YOUR EYES

BO1X ▸ He says that by right of birth, all the gifts of the world are yours to give so you may bring a drop of clarity to those without light.

BO1X ▸ He says "My Spirit of Delight."

BO3X ▸ Feel, sense, and live ancestors running in your being.

BO1X ▸ Dive down into this foundation and reach the Spirit of Delight.

BO3X ▸ Come up to the surface and see yourself bound with beams of light, breathing love and accomplishment onto your skin.

ROUND MIRROR

BO3X ▸ See yourself as a perfectly polished, round mirror.

BO1X ▸ See the soul of your heart reflected clearly as a sunny orb. Then see the soul of your heart reflected clearly as a fountain flowing and outpouring the starry sands of creation.

BO3X ▸ See now in one grain of this sand all the heavens.

BO1X ▸ See in a drop of light all the universe.

BO3X ▸ See yourself now as round, then as a flying, round bird, soaring from star-to- star singing. What do you experience?

MY SOUL'S PROGRESS

BO3X ▸ See the darkened garment that has obscured your being burned and consumed.

BO1X ▸ See now under it, the pearl of all beauty.

OPEN AND RE-CLOSE YOUR EYES

BO3X ▸ See how the flame of desire has destroyed your body and see how the flame of faith is embracing your soul. See the soul becoming clear light, returning to light.

BO1X ▸ Become new, transforming and transfiguring.

BO1X ▸ See yourself enlarged and then like a dot, nearly disappearing into an explosion of the brightest light that is named Truth. What do you experience?

JEWEL OF THE NIGHT

BO3X ▸ See yourself floating as a cloud. Blue stars are crossing you. Slide to this new point, where you and I are joining freely. Be in joy as a jeweled part of the shining sky thrown among the jewels of this radiant sea.

SPRINGING ABOVE

BO3X ▸ See and know that improvement is in the future. It doesn't exist now.

BO1X ▸ Know that if you need the realization of being saved, separate now from those you love, all of them being on their way.

BO1X ▸ Be alone now and know how to spring and soar swiftly. What happens?

ONE DAY THE MESSIAH WILL COME

BO3X ▸ Be waiting for the Messiah. You soul-waiting is concealed in the heights into the Highest Soul. Wait for the Messiah in this blooming crown of life.

BO1X ▸ See yourself traveling on all nuances of the rainbow, refining the colored lights of your being waiting for the Messiah to come.

BO3X ▸ See yourself now made of white light, living into this Highest Soul, waiting…

BO1X ▸ For the Messiah to come. What happens?

THE BEING OF LIGHT

BO3X ▸ See and experience the appearance of perfect nature coming with triumph, glory, knowledge, beauty, grace, and purity.

BO1X ▸ Know now that you are wanting God. Give thanks to be.

THE LOVE OF MY BEING

BO3X ► Know and live how "I love and I am more"; then know and live, "I am not." Know where this ambiguity comes from.

BO3X ► See the love of your being as light – all pervading, clear, blue-white light; light of life self-contained in the core; dense, starry, the true Milky Way, this love of my Being.

WITH A TWINKLE

BO3X ► See a twinkle in your eye. Now send a glance to the Absolute, throw sparks from your heart. See the Absolute now pour on you the radiant flow of life. See yourself shining.

PRAYER: PUTTING YOURSELF IN GOD'S HANDS

BO3X ► See, sense, feel, and live yourself as infinite in space and time.

BO1X ► Feel free to find in everyone the perfect image to contemplate.

BO1X ► Ask God for the "right thing" to be done. Put it in God's hands for His Will to be.

IN ETERNITY

BO3X ► See, sense, and feel reaching Absolute Bliss. Sense time and the need for time to vanish from your mind.

BO1X ► Know in this instant you and God are eternal.

DIVINATION

BO3X ▸ Find the Divine in all that is and exists.

OPEN YOUR EYES AND RE-CLOSE THEM

BO3X ▸ Live the State of Grace behind appearance.

OPEN AND RE-CLOSE YOUR EYES

BO3X ▸ Know how by turning your senses inward and by sensuous sharing, you reach the core. Accept this exact place in the world that we all have by birth.

OPEN AND RE-CLOSE YOUR EYES

BO3X ▸ Feel in your soul a spark of the world soul. Feel and know your eyes becoming the windows of your soul.

EATING THE MENU INSTEAD OF THE MEAL

BO3X ▸ See and know how living in illusion is to be cut from reality.

BO3X ▸ See, know, and sense how the mind is a reality that can change the world. See it changing you.

CREATION ▸ WITHOUT BEGINNING OR END, WE CREATE

BO3X ▸ See and live how you are changing all the time.

BO1X ▸ See and know how every existing thing is changing, too.

BO1X ▸ Know how through this changing, we really depend on each other.

OPEN YOUR EYES.

BO3X ▸ See, feel, and live that God has created us and we constantly recreate God.

BO1X ▸ Know that without beginning, without end, we create.

UNBOUNDED

BO3X ▸ Cast away your little self. In the space that is made, is God.

BO1X ▸ Face God when He enters.

BO1X ▸ Feel God's Omnipresence, ever present to you.

OPEN YOUR EYES AND RE-CLOSE THEM

BO3X ▸ Now know freedom. Have nothing to fear and nothing to gain. What do you feel?

OPEN YOUR EYES

If you feel joy, then CLOSE YOUR EYES AND BO3X ▸ Feel this unbounded joy then feel yourself unbounded.

NO SEPARATION

BO3X ▸ See, feel, and know that as much as you need God, God needs you.

BO1X ▸ Express this no-separation as oneness. Become a point, increasing in unlimited space. (Everywhere and everything.)

BO1X ▸ Feel and live that in the here and now You are me.

UNBROKEN WHOLENESS

BO3X ▸ See yourself immersing into the sea, but not disappearing. Feel one with the whole. Feel one and complete.

BO3X ▸ See yourself added to the eternal soul, linked now with all souls. Feel yourself living.

THE ONLY MIND

BO3X ▸ See yourself constructing the world in the same way as God, then go from multiplicity to Oneness.

BO1X ► Become united with the One and experience your mind as the One Mind.

NON-DUAL

BO3X ► See and know that in being part of The One, there is no more the non-dual duality parting the unity.

BO1X ► Know that you are the One, no longer an outsider, helping to be the complete Universal Absolute One.

KNOWING

BO3X ► Know, see, and live that totality is you. Know how you are infinite, immortal, new forever.

TRANSPOSITION

BO3X ► See, sense, and feel yourself residing in the totality of Being, returning to yourself with reverence.

BO1X ► Be bending now in front of every creature and give thanks.

THE LIVING GOD

BO3X ► See the Living God in nine mirrors reflected through the Tree of Life.

BO1X ► See and sense the Vital Force channeled there and then pour it on every living being for us to know and learn.

BO1X ▸ See the Living God on your breast from and by the Sacred Source of Creation.

CLOSER

BO3X ▸ See yourself diving deeper and deeper into the deepest of being, encompassing all creation.

BO1X ▸ Be in the bottom of the water, entering by silent contact, in dread and shame, with what you know is Absolute.

KISS OF LIFE

BO3X ▸ Be waiting night and day for God to give the Kiss of Life.

BO1X ▸ Feel the enchantment and perfect love capturing you in a rapture that recreates this "I" night and day.

BO1X ▸ Now see each of the things that have caused you pain and release them to the heavens.

BO1X ▸ Bring down from heaven all you need for health, happiness, love, well-being, and prosperity. See them as colors moving toward you. Capture for a moment the color you are most attracted to and discover which of your needs it represents. Know you will draw this into your life.

Self Renewal

"Doors of perception of the Senses, bringing Beauty,
Energy, Love and Ecstasy."
-Colette, "Doors of Perception"

GLOBAL RENEWAL

BO3X ► See the people of the world passing over the abyss by building bridges over the chasms of contradictions. Build a bridge across your own chasm of contradiction.

BO3X ► See and sense all people leaving behind their hatred and violence as they cross the binding bridges of peace and cooperation.

BO1X ► Do the same for yourself or for a special circumstance concerning you.

BO3X ► See and feel all the contradictions in yourself and others being brought into a harmonious brotherhood, all people meeting together on the other side of the abyss. What do you experience?

BO3X ► See and imagine abundance for all springing from the depths of the worldwide fertile earth, giving food, shelter, and security for all, including yourself.

BO3X ► See all the people of the earth living in Eden.

BO3X ► See, sense, feel, know, and live yourself and all humankind becoming a child of God, a student of God, an example of God, an instrument of God.

....

HEALING BY SELF-ORGANIZING

BO3X ► See yourself continually reorganizing your dissipating energy to maintain or increase internal self-order.

BO3X ► See a fracture healing.

BO1X ► See a wound healing.

BO1X ► See an immunological response.

BO1X ► See them all as self-organizing processes that establish order amid disorder.

BO3X ► See and feel fever as aiding to overcome disease.

BO1X ► Feel, sense, and see heat in the area of a healing wound.

BO3X ► See yourself generating thermal heat on some part of your body.

BO1X ► See yourself like a classical healer, placing your hands over a wounded place on someone's body, helping them generate their own heat.

BO3X ► Sift through a basket of seeds, finding some that are not good. Take them out and burn them. Look at the burnt seeds, plant them, and watch them attentively.

BO3X ► Feel and sense how your hand temperature has to remain constant while healing yourself or others.

BO3X ► Sense, feel, and know how you are bringing or helping the possibility of an increased ordering of the system by concentrating the thought, will, and energy on the point you are seeing.

BO3X ► Imagine entering your own body and traveling to the spot that is hurting. Take the time to travel. When you arrive at the spot, look at some warm, soothing oil and imagine pouring it over the spot. Imagine the warm, bright liquid on the spot. See and feel its good effects. See how the warm, bright oil is curing.

BO5X ► With a lasso or a belt, circle the place containing the pain. Tie it up, then release it by throwing the lasso or belt away to the left or to the back.

BO3X ► See a mirror. Write around it about an old remorse. Then see into the mirror how this old thought had occurred. Live all the old feelings and now erase all the remorse-images to the left.

BO1X ▸ Turn over the mirror and in this other face do an opposite act about something glad or happy. See and feel how illuminating is our power in front of ourselves.

BO3X ▸ See in front of you a scale with two balance pans. On the central rod, engrave the words good, perfect, and immutable. Then see how each act or desire to do has the right weight, so no act or desire is offensive.

FROM TWILIGHT TO RAINBOW: HEALING UNCERTAINTY

BO3X ▸ Look at the twilight until the total disappearance of the sun beneath the hill.

BO1X ▸ Sense and feel the difference in your emotions.

BO3X ▸ Look at the twilight until the total disappearance of the sun. Find in you a place that you enjoy. Sense and feel the difference in your emotions.

BO3X ▸ Look at the multi-colored twilight when the sun is sinking at the horizon of the sea. How are you reacting? What do you feel?

BO3X ▸ Imagine you are in front of a threshold. How do you cross it? What do you do? Are you jumping over it, crossing it quickly, standing without moving?

BO3X ▸ See yourself as the hero crossing the threshold over the edge of a radiant sword.

BO1X ▸ See and know that you are between one state and another. Feel the uncertainty and the ambivalence inhabiting you. Describe them.

BO1X ▸ See and live the ending of one sort of life and the beginning of another as entering a new cycle.

THE MYTHS WE LIVE AND DIE BY: FROM SAM KEEN*

Note: A medical doctor who was a healthcare specialist at destroying myths, made me see dealing with disease as passing by three stages:

BO3X ▸ The "I/it" stage, where we fear we are the victim of germs, heredity, environment, etc., so we are helpless and not responsible. We need an outside agent to heal us. Destroy that myth.

BO1X ▸ The "I/Thou" stage, when we begin to talk to the disease and realize all is connected to us and in our life.

BO1X ▸ The "I/I" stage, when by listening to the voice of the pain and not resisting it, we cut the quantity of the pain. The body is trying to say to us through the disease, "We have to speak to the disease as to a child, firmly, but reassuring it of something."

FINISHING WITH THE PAST

BO1X ▸ Sense memories on your skin. Sense how event after event, place after place, emotion after emotion is coming out of your skin. Each time something comes out, imagine rubbing your skin by massaging outward, circulating whatever stays on the skin of the special memory.

THE LIFE CYCLE OF A BUD

BO3X ▸ See yourself lying down, getting in touch with how your body feels.

BO1X ▸ Now imagine that your left hand is a small flower bud, which slowly grows and moves toward the sunlight. Your flower slowly opens its petals to the breeze and opens to the light rain, whose sound is accompanying its movement.

BO1X ▸ Now feel what your flower energy is giving to the forming of the seeds. See the flower withering. See it gradually sink down to the ground with its seeds.

BO1X ▸ You are a seed again. Keep your body in a closed position. What kind of a seed are you?

BO1X ▸ It is springtime and you begin to sprout and move, sending a small root into the soil and a small shoot toward the sunlight…

BO1X ▸ and continue to grow and move, becoming aware of how your body feels as you slowly unfold from your seed and grow into a plant or tree.

IMMORTALITY FATAL, FATAL IMMORTALITY

BO7X ▸ WHILE COUNTING BACKWARDS FROM 7 TO 1, WITH AN OUT-BREATH ON EACH NUMBER. SEE EACH NUMBER CLEARLY, ESPECIALLY NUMBER "1".

BO1X ▸ See a screen. On the screen see and know how what you sow you must harvest.

BO7X ▸ COUNTING BACKWARDS FROM 7 TO 1, WITH AN OUT-BREATH ON EACH NUMBER — Imagine You have a glass of clear seltzer. Drink it slowly. See and feel seven bubbles. Push away the bubbles and enter one of them. Follow the other six bubbles. What is happening?

BO7X ▸ WHILE COUNTING BACKWARDS FROM 7 TO 1, WITH AN OUT-BREATH ON EACH NUMBER — See seven seeds.

BO7X ▸ COUNTING BACKWARDS FROM 7 TO 1, WITH AN OUT-BREATH ON EACH NUMBER — Imagine seven crosses. Describe what is happening.

BO1X ▸ WHILE COUNTING BACKWARDS FROM 7 TO 1, WITH AN OUT-BREATH ON EACH NUMBER — See seven postcards quickly. Describe them.

BO1X ▸ WHILE COUNTING BACKWARDS FROM 7 TO 1, WITH AN OUT-BREATH ON EACH NUMBER — See a wall of seven doors. Choose one and open it. Describe it.

BO3X ▸ You are at a labyrinth. There is a crossway and seven paths. Choose and follow a path. When you reach the end, come back by the same path to the crossway. Describe the path.

BO3X ▸ You are on a distressed boat. There are seven people and only one safety belt. What is happening?

BO3X ▸ You are standing in the middle of an earthquake. Take seven people out of danger. Describe them.

BO7X ▸ COUNTING BACKWARDS FROM 7 TO 1, WITH AN OUT-BREATH ON EACH NUMBER – Onto a screen see seven fish. Describe them.

Bring Above Below Together
to Unite Differences

"In the abyss of the unknown are hidden hideous monsters —
…Calm and quiet, I wait for those that are just there. Then they
transform…ready for the quest of the sweet soft hidden princess."
-Colette, "The Green Lion Swallows the Sun"

DESCENT INTO SELF, THE BOTTOMLESS ABYSS: FROM PIERRE TEILHARD DE CHARDIN*

BO3X ▸ Take a lamp and leave the zone of everyday preoccupation and relationships, where everything seems clear.

BO1X ▸ With your lamp, go down a staircase, taking a breath out at every step. At the bottom, see a new person waiting there for you and ask its name.

BO1X ▸ Go to your innermost self, reaching the deep abyss where you feel deeply that your power of action emanates.

BO1X ▸ Sense and feel what it is like to go farther and farther from conventional certainties by which your social life is made up.

BO1X ▸ Sense how easy it is to lose contact with your self. Stay conscious and cautious.

BO1X ▸ See and feel that at each step of the descent a new person is disclosed in you. See them clearly and try to know their names. If the name is not coming easily, ask for it.

BO1X ▸ Sense how without finding its name, the new being is no longer obeying you.

BO1X ▸ Stop your exploration when your path has disappeared or faded under your feet.

BO1X ▸ See that there is a bottomless abyss out of which is arising what is really your life. Sense it, feel it, recognize it, and know how to contact it, when necessary. Be sure to remember all that.

BO3X ▸ Return to your everyday life by climbing up each step and recognizing each of your selves. Every time you return to see one of your selves, recognize the power of action attached to it.

BO1X ▸ Look again at the bottomless abyss and at each of your selves.

BO1X ▸ OPEN YOUR EYES and imagine you can reach this place and these beings very fast. Sense and know how every time you want to reach them, you may obtain the best of what they give you in knowledge and in power of action.

BO3X ▸ See and sense how by curtailing your spontaneity you may lose richness and expansion of energy.

BO3X ▸ Sense the physical exertion connected with the preoccupation of your emotional and mental safety.

BO1X ▸ Looking into a mirror, notice that as you are withholding your secret, you are suffering from shallow breathing.

BO3X ▸ Feel and know how by becoming self-awakening you prevent yourself from falling into these errors by permitting you to meet with yourself.

....

ASCENT: FROM EINSTEIN

BO3X ▸ See and know how unity and universality are not mutually exclusive values, but are two sides of the same reality, compensating, fulfilling, and complementing each other.

BO3X ▸ See how they are becoming one in the experience of enlightenment.

BO1X ▸ See how this experience does not dissolve the mind into an amorphous all.

BO3X ▸ Realize that the individual itself contains totality focalized in your very core.

BO3X ▸ Sense, as many physicists have, that the distinctions between past, present, and future are all an illusion.

BO3X ▸ Feel this unmistakable intimation of immortality.

BO3X ▸ Sense and know with Einstein that this is the whole and this is immortality.

BO3X ► See how reality, including time, persons, life, and death, is not what we have taken it to be.

THE FOAM AND THE SEA: FROM EINSTEIN

BO3X ► See the sea becoming calm and flat. The foam sparkles with the reflected light of the sun. Enter the water and swim to the horizon, to the place between the sky and the water. See, sense, and feel what happens to you between the sky and water as they enter you from above and below. Then, come back to the shore on your back, backstroking. Now on the beach, kneel down and take a handful of sand. Let it sift through your fingers until one grain is left in your palm. Look at it until it forms into something.

BO3X ► Enter the ocean, swimming between the blue and white color of the ocean water.

BO3X ► Walking along the water's edge, enter the water. Diving in, find a grotto beneath the surface. Enter the grotto and meet your ancestor or ancestors. Hear what they have to tell you. Thank them and swim back to shore on top of the foam, which you feel above and beneath you.

TO KNOW YOUR CREATION

BO3X ► See and know how your righteous deeds bring you to wholeness.

BO1X ► See how this wholeness branches into your creations. See and know what these creations become.

RELEASING EVIL TO CREATE WHOLENESS: FROM *THE BOOK OF ADAM*

"In the name of Sovereign Life Over Life, be helping me."

BO3X ▸ Keeping that in mind, review the emotional and physical disturbances that have been in your past. Then...

BO3X ▸ See yourself as a tree shaken by the Hand of God. See and sense that the bark is falling from you. This bark becomes fertilizer in the earth. See the insects living under the bark, then falling down and disappearing into the earth. Sense and see the place of the malaise or disease, discomfort, discord, or in-completion becoming larger spaces where discomfort, discord, or incompletion is diluted by light.

BO1X ▸ See and sense the dilution until light is filling every place and all the space.

BO1X ▸ See all evil going out of your skin and mouth as a light smoke.

Note: Do the following exercise every morning for 7 days.

BO3X ▸ See yourself parted into many different pieces. Put them together into one united being.

BO1X ▸ See and feel the borders between the different pieces slowly disappearing as you become one.

BO3X ▸ Make an ointment of sky and sun and spread it on a wound, which be-comes normal skin.

....

THE ABYSS OF MYSTERY — THE GIFT OF WONDER: FROM EINSTEIN

BO3X ▸ Feel and know how what you experience as mysterious is not the feared, but the beautiful in you.

BO3X ▸ Feel and know this abyss of mystery and wonder.

BO3X ► See and know that this abyss brings you to the fundamental cradle of the true self, art, science, and every discovery.

BO3X ► See and sense how this abyss of mystery and wonder is opening our dimmed eyes to the marvel in us.

BO3X ► Sense and see how in this abyss you are aware of what is in you.

BO3X ► See and feel how revealing this hidden thing is bringing an unimaginable surprise.

BO3X ► See and know how the list of our actions resounds down to infinite depths.

BO1X ► Hear this resounding and know quickly how every time you choose to reach your list of actions, you may obtain the best of what it may give you in power of action and knowledge.

BO1X ► Thank all that is in you and return peacefully to your everyday life in clarity.

BO1X AND WITH OPEN EYES sense how enriched you are and feel renewed.

BO1X ► Make nine decisions now for the near future [three months].

....

FROM BACHYA BEN JOSEPH IBN PAKUDA*

BO3X ► See now and know forever that your true guide is the Image of God in you.

BO1X ► Looking at others in a state of contemplation, see every creature as created by God or in the Image of God.

BO3X ► Turning your head 180 degrees and telling the truth, know how to live with humility and to sense it as a gift in the other and in yourself.

BO1X ► Live the purest love until its peak.

BO1X ► Return to the beginning of the pure feeling and repair something that you must.

BO3X ▸ Now that you have repaired something, you have to repent. Do it by reversing your perspective, your attitude, your actions. Be conscious of any change in yourself.

....

TO MEET WITH YOURSELF:
FROM BACHYA BEN JOSEPH IBN PAKUDA

BO3X ▸ Look into a screen to see how you function best.

BO1X ▸ Now look into the screen when all aspects of yourself are integrated.

BO1X ▸ See the physical basis well in place and sustaining the play of a strong emotion.

BO1X ▸ See and know how your mind is helping your body keep the suitable balance.

BO3X ▸ See and feel into a mirror how to grow. Be totally honest with yourself and look at your face. Recognize it.

BO3X ▸ See into a mirror and sense the necessity to be completely open.

BO1X ▸ Imagine now that you keep a secret. Then into a mirror look at your tightened body.

BO1X ▸ Sense the necessary vigilance and suspicion that is hardening your face.

BO3X ▸ Live and know how each little anger or dispute is an opportunity to see how we can liberate ourselves from our love of imposed self-constraint on the other or others.

BO1X ▸ See and feel how our chance to change and maintain health is in our ability to change.

Healing Through Science

"In the transparent empty space He resides,
In vibrant clear Light and tranquil harmony."
-Colette, "The Only One"

PRAYERS FOR PEACE: FROM EZEKIEL

BO3X ▶ See the likeness of the speaking silence.

BO1X ▶ What is the speaking silence telling you?

BO1X ▶ Know who is the you to whom the speaking silence is speaking.

SILENCE: FROM *THE BOOK OF ADAM*

BO3X ▶ Hear and sense the life in yourself being the helper of your life.

BO3X ▶ See, feel, and know how by looking through the window to the inside, you are the guardian of yourself.

BO3X ▶ See, feel, and know how by watching the outside, you are the guardian of your brother.

BO3X ▶ See, feel, and know how the only praise worthy of You the Almighty is silence. With this awareness, Divine Mercy does not cease to descend on you.

FROM TAOISM

BO1X ▶ Close your eyes and you will see clarity. Cease to listen and you will hear truth. Be silent and your heart will sing.

BO1X ► Seek no contact and you will find union. Be still and you will move forward on the tide of the Spirit. Be gentle with reverence and you will need no strength.

BO1X ► Be patient and you will achieve all things. Remember not to hurry and not to worry.

BO1X ► Be humble and you will remain entire.

BO1X ► Take no heed of time and apply.

THE WAY OF QUIESCENCE: FROM TAOISM

BO1X ► Turn your concentration to your entire being. Enter the inside.

BO1X ► Sense your concentration continuing effortlessly.

BO1X ► Your concentration becomes calm without effort.

BO1X ► Calm without effort becomes firm and stable.

SONGS OF KABIR*
TRANSLATED BY RABINDRANATH TAGORE*

BO3X ► Hear to what shore you did cross, oh my heart.
There is no traveler before you.
There is no road; there is no water; there is no boat.
No boatman is there.
There is not so much as a rope to tow the boat or a man to draw it.
No earth; no sky.
Nothing is there.
No fjord, no shore.

BO1X ► Here there is neither body nor mind, and you shall find naught in your emptiness.

BO1X ► Be strong and enter into your body, for there your foothold is firm.

BO3X ► See, sense, feel, and live:
Consider it well, oh my heart.
Go not elsewhere.
Put all thought away and stand fast in that which you are.

BO3X ► Hear, oh my heart.
    You have not known of the secrets of the city of love.

BO3X ► See, feel, and know that in ignorance you came and in ignorance you return and there is never moonlight and never dark.

BO3X ► See by what this land is illuminated—
    The rays of millions of suns.

THE SUFI WAY

BO3X ► Know that the universe is a large human being. See that man is a little universe.

BO1X ► Know and live why it has been told, "Be the child of the moment."

BO3X ► See a djinni* (genie) swallowing you. How do you feel?

BO1X ► See yourself swallowing the djinni. What happens?

BO3X ► Live and know that from god to god, there is nothing else than God.

BO3X ► Know what it is to live into the Garden of Piety.

BO1X ► Don't stay on the shore, but fight against the tide.

BO1X ► Know and live that the heart of the believer is the highest sky.

BO1X ► Know and live that the whole earth is a mosque.

BO3X ► When the soul has received the seed from the soul, by this soul the world is.

BO1X ► Live and know why "The hidden treasure is a jar full of wisdom and beauty."

Embryo of Immortality

"I reach Absolute bliss.
When Time is vanishing from the Mind…"
-Colette, "In the Eternity, Now"

STRESS WITHOUT DISTRESS

BO3X ▸ See in front of you an abyss. There is no bridge to cross over and no sword on which to cross over.

BO1X ▸ See yourself now wearing a bright turban. Feel the courage, the decision, and the energy to jump over the abyss.

BO3X ▸ Know and feel being at the same time dark and light.

BO3X ▸ See and feel being at the same time heaven and earth.

BO3X ▸ See and sense how pleasure, challenges, achievement, and fulfillment are other forms of stress.

BO3X ▸ See and sense how distress comes from repeated assaults on the nervous system.

BO3X ▸ See how you have to mobilize in people the will to be healed.

BO1X ▸ See how you have to want to cure.

BO3X ▸ See how aiming toward wellness through imagery is bringing balance and synchronization between one's inner and outer self.

BO1X ▸ See how you are creating a clear idea of what is desired and the possibilities to obtain it.

EXISTING IS RESISTING

BO3X ► See stress as any condition that damages or disturbs the body, causing breakdown, crying, or the death of a few or many cells.

BO3X ► See and live stress as the weight of the wear and tear of fear caused by living.

BO3X ► Sense how your body is reacting when cutting your finger, when hearing disturbing noises, or having a picnic.

BO3X ► See and live how your nervous system is sending an SOS to your body's messengers, the hormones, which quickly go into action.

BO3X ► See and sense how in response to the alarm signal, special hormones rush to the injured area, where they steady the work of the healing process.

BO3X ► See how hormones speed up or slow down activity when needed.

BO1X ► See and sense how they are helping by resisting disease and healing injury.

BO3X ► See how as the hormones are working, your body goes into a natural order of working.

BO3X ► See and sense how well your body is handling many frequent stressful experiences and how well you are resisting them.

BO3X ► See and sense how you may avoid being hurt by excessive stress. Find your own way.

BO3X ► See and live how your body is embodied thoughts, sensations, images, and light.

RELAX TO UNSTRESS

BO3X ▸ See how under stress your body is reacting as your mind.

BO3X ▸ See how to be healthy you have to reach a wholeness with all functions of body and mind becoming normally active.

BO1X ▸ Sense this state of complete physical, mental, and social well-being.

BO3X ▸ See how health is not measured by the absence of disease or infirmity.

BO1X ▸ Sense how health is the measure of how much energy the organism has to cope with the environment.

BO3X ▸ See and live how health is a state of mind permitting your body to relax and stand out of the way.

BO1X ▸ See how when using imagery to relax, you avoid setting up roadblocks— and see that Nature can heal us and maintain homeostasis

BO3X ▸ See and sense how Nature brings internal stability through the coordinated responses of the different parts of the body, mind, and emotions.

....

THE NEW YEAR OF THE TREE

BO3X ▸ Recognize the most important task you have accomplished in the past year. Ask yourself how you are expressing this actual task through your body.

BO1X ▸ Feel like a tree. Sense your feet going down to the earth. Sense your hands going up toward heaven. Feel pulled in different directions yet at the same time attuned with all of them.

BO1X ▸ Feel your body as one and start dancing.

TIME PRESSURE: PRESSED FOR TIME

BO3X ▸ See and sense yourself being pressed for time.

BO1X ▸ Sense and know being pressed for time is really being pressed by time.

BO1X ▸ Remove the pressure of time by decompressing your relationship with time. Know now that you control your own time.

RELAX TO UNDO

BO3X ▸ See and live how health is a state of mind that permits the body to be relaxed and avoid deterioration.

BO3X ▸ See and feel your anus muscle at the floor of your pelvis. Note how it looks. See and sense the muscle being stretched and elongated until it is free of constriction.

BO1X ▸ Know that you can stretch and elongate you anus muscle whenever it constricts by using this exercise. See and feel the anus muscle at the floor of your pelvis soothed and relaxed. Now see a pair of golden hands stretching and elongating this muscle until it releases its constriction.

BO1X ▸ Know that when this muscle contracts, you can elongate it, freeing yourself of pain and restriction.

ERROR BECOMING WONDER

BO3X ▸ See how the image of movement is the active motion of physical movement and sports.

BO3X ▸ See how the error of immobility may be moved by Imagery.

BO1X ▸ See how restlessness is a mind attitude.

BO1X ▸ See how Imagery is exercise oriented.

BO3X ▸ See and sense how exercising is a factor of vitality and health.

BO1X ▸ See yourself imaging circulation and notice how imaging is improving it. See your activated circulation regulating the movements of stomach, lungs, and heart.

BO1X ▸ See how images are facilitating and regulating activity, improving diseases caused by inactivity, mobilizing the immune system, and resisting infection by the production of anti-bodies.

GUILT, REPETITION AND TRUTH

BO3X ▸ See and feel that guilt is the very nerve of sorrow.

BO2X ▸ See and know how through depression and sadness someone can forget who they really are.

BO1X ▸ Know and recognize that everything depends on truth. Know that if you are becoming depressed, it is because of a lack of truth and you must begin anew.

BO1X ▸ See, sense, and know that if you are not finding the truth, you may begin again as if for the first time.

ONENESS WITH THE UNIVERSE: FROM EINSTEIN

BO3X ▸ See, sense, and know that the individual itself contains the totality.

BO3X ▸ See, sense, feel, and know how our essential oneness with the universe is in sameness or unqualified identity.

BO1X ▸ See, sense, feel, and know that it is an organic relationship.

BO3X ▸ See how differentiation and uniqueness of function are as important as ultimate and basic unity.

Seeking Truth The Eastern Way

"Tied up to the Ultimate but Immanent reality
My being depends on the Invisible."
-Colette, "Moi, Bienheureuse Infortunée!"

LAO TZU*, FOUNDER OF TAOISM

BO3X ► Live how kindness in words creates confidence.

BO3X ► Live how kindness in thinking creates profundity and depth.

BO1X ► Live how kindness in giving creates love.

....

THE *TAO TEH CHING*: BY LAO TZU

BO3X ► Find and live that whoever knows their light and stays in their shadow is the model, pattern, and mirror of the world.

BO3X ► Feel and live how this is the opposite of the western view "For whom to put his or her life under wood is a sin." [i.e. hiding your light under a bushel]

....

CHINESE EDUCATION ► FROM *TAO TEH CHING*: BY LAO TZU

BO3X ► See yourself sitting still. Know how if you are not doing that, you are half developed. Know that by feeling how it is to sit still, you are enjoying totally.

BO3X ▸ See yourself in three mirrors as a stupid one arguing, as the talented one talking, as the sage not speaking and enjoying it.

BO3X ▸ See yourself as a teacher having to teach children without writing, reading, or telling them how to behave or what to do.

BO1X ▸ Know why the really great teachers have never written their teachings.

BO3X ▸ Feel and know how "you are the way." See and recognize someone you love being for him or her "the way."

BO3X ▸ Feel and know how by transmission, the merits of the father and the mother are in you. See yourself sharing the merits with someone you love. Then see yourself sharing the merits with someone you want to help. What do you do and how do you feel?

BO3X ▸ Feel and know how you are separate from each other even if you want to be united to each other.

BO1X ▸ Feel how love is the only cohesive element.

BO3X ▸ Know that life is a process of self-realization.

BO1X ▸ Recognize how you are becoming, how you are, and becoming who you are.

BO1X ▸ Know how you become what you are only by direct experience.

BO3X ▸ See and know how you are discovering by yourself all that is valuable.

BO3X ▸ Live and know how by accepting consciousness of self you are entering the wheel of becoming.

BO1X ▸ Know and feel how Nirvana is living an immediate becoming.

BO3X ▸ Feel how you are brothers and sisters with others whether or not someone else knows it.

BO1X ▸ Feel and live yourself sharing the essence of life with all forms of life.

WATER AS PRECEPTOR ▸ FROM THE *TAO TEH CHING*: BY LAO TZU

BO3X ▸ See and sense yourself as water washing away and giving contour to rocks.

BO1X ▸ See and sense yourself as water corroding iron until it crumbles to dust.

BO1X ▸ See and sense yourself as water saturating the atmosphere as the winds direct you to the sea. Know that water yields to obstacles with deceptive humility.

WATER AS PRECEPTOR, WATER TO FLOWER ▸ FROM THE *TAO TEH CHING*: BY LAO TZU

BO3X ▸ Sensing that the power of water may prevent you from following its destined course to the sea…

BO3X ▸ … see and know as water how by yielding and by not attacking, you always conquer and win the battle.

BO3X ▸ See, sense, feel, live, and know yourself as the sage, how making yourself as water you become distinguished for your humility.

BO1X ▸ See, sense, feel, live, and know yourself as the sage embodying a deep calmness.

BO1X ▸ See, sense, feel, live, and know how acting from non-action, the sage conquers the world.

Between Life and Death Choose Life

"Don't succumb if success is not yet answering,
See it here and now. It will be, for it is."
-Colette, "In A Moment of Triumph"

STAIRCASE OF CLOUDS

BO3X ▸ See yourself walking very slowly at dusk on a staircase of clouds.

BO3X ▸ See yourself at the end of the day, going farther and farther, climbing higher and higher.

BO3X ▸ Imagine yourself disappearing beyond the clouds.

BO3X ▸ Sense how between night and day the disappearance is natural and normal.

BO3X ▸ Sense how this disappearance is a form of death.

BO1X ▸ See yourself between life and death.

BO1X ▸ Choose life and tell yourself the reasons.

BO3X ▸ Look at a metallic tube.

BO1X ▸ Look at a gong made of a tree trunk hitting the metallic tube.

BO1X ▸ Hear the vibrating and resounding.

BO3X ▸ Look at a metallic tube hitting a gong made of a tree trunk.

BO1X ▸ Hear the vibrating and resounding for the liberation of the birds in the air.

BO1X ▸ Hear the vibrating and resounding for the liberation of the soul.

BO3X ▸ Hear how the early bird catches the entire world.

DESCENT INTO THE SELF

BO3X ► Imagine that you take a lamp and leave the zone of everyday preoccupation, occupation, and relationship, where everything seems clear.

BO1X ► With a lamp, go down to your innermost self.

BO1X ► At every step, see the new person you are and ask their name.

BO3X ► Reach the deep abyss, where you feel how deeply your power of action emanates.

BO3X ► Sense and feel how it is to move further and further from conventional certainty by which your social life is developed.

BO1X ► Sense how easy it is to lose contact with this new freedom.

BO1X ► Stay conscious and cautious.

BO3X ► See how with each step of the descent, a new person is disclosed in you. See them clearly.

BO1X ► Try to know their name.

BO1X ► Sense how without your finding its name, this person no longer obeys you.

BO3X ► Stop your exploration only when the path has disappeared or faded under your feet.

BO1X ► See how there is a bottomless abyss out of which is arising what is really your life.

BO3X ► Return to your everyday life, climbing up to the light. At each step recognize each of your selves and the power of action attached to them.

BO1X ► OPEN YOUR EYES SLOWLY. Looking again into the bottomless abyss, see each of yourselves. Imagine you may very quickly reach your power of action at this place within.

....

LIVING AT THE EDGE OF A KNIFE

BO3X ► See yourself living dangerously.

BO3X ► See and live every dangerous moment of your life from the earliest to the most current time.

BO1X ▸ At each instance ask yourself if you want to retain the moment.

BO1X ▸ Hear what the moment is telling you.

BO3X ▸ Return to every dangerous moment starting now and going in reverse, seeking to know what each moment taught you at the time and what it is teaching you now.

TAKING LIFE ON THE GOOD SIDE

BO3X ▸ See yourself going forward. What do you feel?

BO1X ▸ See yourself going to the right. What do you feel?

BO1X ▸ See yourself going to the left. What do you feel?

BO1X ▸ See yourself going upward. What do you feel?

BO1X ▸ See yourself going downward. What do you feel?

BO1X ▸ What have you understood?

BO3X ▸ See yourself inspire and breathe life sweetly.

BO1X ▸ See yourself living happily with all your being.

BO3X ▸ Imagine that the ground under your hand is silk paper on which advice is written. What is it?

BO3X ▸ See yourself on a slide plunging into a pool and find something of yours which is lost or forgotten.

BO3X ▸ See yourself seated on a banister that you can slide down.

BO1X ▸ Make your arm longer as you are trying to find something that is there for you.

BO3X ▸ See and know that the answer is in the basement. Descend on an elevator to find the answer.

PROMPTNESS URGE

BO3X ▸ Imagine that something unjust has been done to you.

BO1X ▸ Sense your prompting urge calling you for revenge.

BO1X ▸ Feel and see what may be done to gain the revenge.

BO3X ▸ Sense this malicious will telling you that to be vindictive is right and making you strong and proud. What do you feel and know?

BO3X ▸ Find all the ways to hurt and humiliate.

BO1X ▸ Sense that what has been done to you is unforgivable.

BO3X ▸ Sense the bitterness taking possession of you.

BO2X ▸ Sense rancor and resentment inhabiting you.

BO1X ▸ Appreciate their long-lasting company.

BO1X ▸ Sense being aggrieved by some action, person, or finding that makes you spiteful.

BO3X ▸ Meditate on these feelings. Know that if you do not choose to be destroyed by these poisonous emotions, you need to temper and modulate your feelings.

CYCLE OF LIFE AND DEATH

BO3X ▸ See yourself in the womb.

BO1X ▸ See yourself as a newborn.

BO1X ▸ See yourself as an infant.

BO1X ▸ See yourself as a baby.

BO1X ▸ See yourself as a child.

BO1X ▸ See yourself as a teenager.

BO1X ▸ See yourself as a young adult.

BO1X ▸ See yourself as an adult.

BO1X ▸ See yourself as a dead one.

BO1X ▸ See the possibility of being again in the womb, being born and living a new life.

Monotheism: The Passion for Truth

"...My highest soul is kidnapped in its Darkness.
The curtain of Sand-Stars surrounding me
sends Light far behind. On the letters of the High,
waiting for me to write the only word, Truth"
-Colette, "Nearer From You"

WARM-UP EXERCISE

BO3X ▸ Know how brain waves in all forms of imagery show an alert state of relaxation, inward attention, and intense creativity.

BO3X ▸ Sense how breathing out permits imagery to be delivered to your consciousness and know how it is a bridge between the visible and invisible worlds.

BO3X ▸ Sense how imagery is a tool to prepare physical and psychological well-being.

BO3X ▸ See and know how awareness of breathing is always at work with imagery.

BO1X ▸ See how centering is always at work with imagery.

BO3X ▸ See and feel how we have only to image to direct energy to the body and to the being.

BO3X ▸ See yourself sitting regularly to image. Imagine you are slowly drinking a glass of water that you feel is a radiant elixir of life, purifying your body and clearing it until it becomes luminescent with perfect health.

JANUS*: DOUBLE FACE, DOUBLE DOOR

BO3X ▸ Live and feel what it is to lose face.

BO1X ▸ Live and feel what it is to put on a long face.

BO1X ▸ Live and feel what it is to be in another's face.

BO1X ▸ In the mirror, see yourself getting free.

BO1X ▸ In the mirror, see yourself painting God's face.

BO1X ▸ In the mirror, see a double-faced God.

BO3X ▸ See and live what it is to be a slave in old Rome. Live the cold and lack of food you have to endure. At the end of the year, beginning in January, see how these conditions we all must endure are a favor, a boon, a lesson.

BO3X ▸ See other people praying to the god Janus with his two faces, one looking at the past, the other at the future.

BO1X ▸ Looking at the double-faced Janus at the end of the past year, the past year beginning yesterday.

BO1X ▸ Look at the nose, mouth, eyes, ears of the double-faced Janus being all open on today and the now. What do you sense and feel when life is coming in by those openings?

BO3X ▸ See the face of Janus looking at the New Year, after seeing and understanding the past year. Now feeling alive, you want to change part of the consequences of the deeds and events of the past year, and have a different attitude toward events and persons in the next year.

BO3X ▸ See yourself double-faced like Janus. Know with Janus' eyes that you see clearly all the necessary changes, the way to make those changes, and what cannot be changed.

SATURN CYCLE: CLEANSING

BO3X ► See how you are weaving your life by replacing in the loom the threads that are not fitting.

BO2X ► See the general colors you are weaving. See the nuances you use for replacing the threads that have been damaged.

BO3X ► Do or undo what is convenient to have the weaving of your choice.

BO3X ► Live how repairing what has been poorly done, at first is rewarding. See how when replacing, your weaving looks and feels new.

BO3X ► See how you are choosing the threads for a new and more beautiful weaving.

BO1X ► Sense and feel how with experience, you are doing what is the best.

BO3X ► Feel and know that if you are really beginning a new weaving, God is preparing the pattern.

SATURNALIA, THE FEAST

BO3X ► See and live as young Janus at the time of the feast of the deity Saturn. Have two days of regrets for your errors and those of others; live three days of change; live and see two days of repentance for excesses, taking and keeping the decision to live a middle way.

BO2X ► See yourself as a slave looking at your master, looking at a judge, looking at an advisor, a teacher, a dictator and choosing who you want to be.

BO1X ► See yourself as a rich master with many slaves, and see yourself a slave for three days. How are you behaving?

SATURN

BO3X ► See during three days all the faces and walls between social levels being abolished.

BO1X ▸ See and live how to throw this out of yourself, the old father dictator, Saturn, requires you to live two days of regrets and three days of change.

BO3X ▸ What are you doing during these three days? What are your sensations and feelings, when changing your life? What is happening to you?

BO3X ▸ Live and see the two following days with the eyes of Janus. See what the New Year is offering. What do you want of it? Try to manage between what you habitually want and your ability to choose change.

BO3X ▸ See and know how your fate has made you a slave, a deported one in Rome, an unaccepted stranger.

BO1X ▸ Sense and know that your soul is free. Feel and know that it is always possible for you to change your fate and to make your destiny.

HOLDING DESTINY IN YOUR HANDS

BO3X ▸ Imagine you are going on a journey on a magic carpet or white cloud. Imagine you are looking down on your house and hometown, seeing some of the people who are important to you. Imagine you are connected to these people by golden strings that permit you to move them and the objects around, as you wish.

BO3X ▸ Imagine now that you are down there included in the scene while at the same time you hold the strings just above.

BO3X ▸ See and sense that we are ready for a mutation or for destruction.

BO3X ▸ See yourself helping by committing yourself to liberate truth.

BO3X ▸ See and feel The Source from where everything is coming.

BO3X ▸ Hear, sense, and see the words of creation being called from The Source.

BO1X ▸ Hear, sense, and see how these words are coming to you. Hear, sense, and feel them clearly and deeply.

BO3X ▸ Sense how with the words of creation your prayer is made.

BO3X ► Hear and follow this prayer, when on its way and returning back to The Source. Hear and sense this flow of creation.

BO3X ► Sense and live how this prayer is joined to the constant flow of Creation.

BO1X ► See, sense and know how you are one with this flow and with the prayer.

THE MAGGID*: ANGEL OF LIGHT

BO3X ► See yourself dreaming a dream of truth for now and foreseeing the future.

BO3X ► Imagine the Prophet Elijah,* the one who never died, revealing himself about your dream of truth.

BO3X ► Imagine the Prophet Elijah again revealing himself about your dream of truth in terms of your faith and your good deeds. Listen respectfully to his advice.

BO3X ► See yourself observing with intention one of the commandments and by this action, seeing an Angel of Light.

CHRISTIANITY: PART I

BO1X ► See and sense that the nature of man is like it is told in the Bible: flesh, soul, and Spirit.

BO3X ► Know that the flesh is more than the body because it also contains biological drives.

BO1X ► Recognize and live the behavior that serves to satiate your appetite.

BO3X ► Know and live how the Spirit is an animating force operating through body and Soul.

BO1X ► Sense and feel the importance of this area of functioning and now that it is there, that God is operating.

BO3X ► See and live how God is experienced existentially and transcendentally by man through his Spirit that lives.

BO1X ► Know that this Spirit lives in the believers in order (1) to reveal truth, (2) to give power, and (3) to fill them through love.

BO3X ► Sense and see how God has given us the power to live according to the values He has given to those in the Bible.

BO3X ► Know how when alienated from God by our own errors, we remain incomplete and long to be whole.

....

CHRISTIANITY: PART II

BO1X ► See and live how health is holiness and wholeness. Sense wholeness as sanctification.

BO3X ► Know how after salvation, man's life is one of constant self-inspection.

BO1X ► Know how to modify the process of self-inspection, you have to live confession, reproof, instruction, and the performance of good work, good will, and love.

BO3X ► See and live how this modifies your behavior, and know how you are becoming whole in body, mind, and Spirit.

BO1X ▸ Have a direct learning. Have a deep insight. Have an immediate experience.

BO1X ▸ Live how when you have reached these inner goals, you are reunited with God and feel completion.

BO1X ▸ See and live how in the Christian way, now is seen as the past and in anticipation of the future.

BO3X ▸ See and live how understanding of the past is indispensable to know and decide what changes may take place and new patterns of behavior be established.

BO1X ▸ Feel and know how emotional knowledge and its understanding are used to help us comprehend our behavior.

BO1X ▸ Feel and know of what use are forgiveness and surrender.

BO1X ▸ Sense and feel how the promise of love, peace, joy, abundance, and eternal life are powerful incentives for forgiveness and surrender.

ISLAM: THERE IS NO GOD BUT GOD

BO2X ▸ Know why "The eye of the sea is not the foam."

BO1X ▸ Forget the foam and look at life with the eye of the sea.

BO2X ▸ See how what is coming from the heart is coming from a window between the heart and the heart.

BO1X ▸ Know how your silence is the decipherer.

BO1X ► Know how your question is the decipherer.

BO2X ► You are not an only you.
You are the highest sky and the deepest sea.
This powerful you is a thousand times like the ocean where are drowned
a hundred like you.

BO2X ► I know God by God, and I know what is not God by God's light.

BO1X ► Live why it is, even though Spirit is always here, we are losing sight of it.

BO1X ► See and know why it is told, "Don't look at the jewels embedded at the
back of the mirror. Look at the polished face of the mirror."

BO1X ► Live and know how to make yourself transparent to the Absolute.

BO1X ► Live and see how if being thirsty you are drinking slowly out of a cup of
water. Know then what is waiting for you into the water.

BO1X ► Know and see how looking at a grain of sand you are looking at the
universe.

The Old Testament

"The Fountain of Wisdom of my ancestors
Is still running in my being."
-Colette, "Fountain of Wisdom"

BO3X ▶ See, sense, live, and feel yourself in the Garden of Your Inner Reality. Become immersed in the fullness of God's truth. Hear the universe echoing Hallelujah. REMEMBER THIS IMAGE AS YOU BREATHE OUT AND OPEN YOUR EYES. SEE THE IMAGE ON THE WALL OPPOSITE YOU AND LET IT FADE AWAY. IF YOU CANNOT SEE IT ON THE WALL, SEE IT IN YOUR MIND'S EYE.

ADAM AND EVE

BO3X ▶ See, sense, and feel God blowing the Breath of Life into you.

BO1X ▶ Know, sense, and see how this breath is the spark that ignites your life force.

BO1X ▶ Feel and see this breath spreading throughout every part of your body, through each organ and cell, filling you with blue/golden light. Know and live how this sparkling health is giving you new life and infusing you with will, joyfulness, and the power to heal.

BO3X ▶ Become Eve being born from the rib of Adam. Know the meaning of the rib as the support of the chest, the place of courage, bravery, and fearlessness. Find this intimacy with Adam.

BO3X ▶ As Adam, be aware of how being united has to give rise to the necessity for two in preparation for giving in to the world of the serpent. Be accepting this reality without sadness.

BO2X ▶ As Eve, see, feel, and sense the power of the serpent's words, promising you to become God. See the Tree of Life and the Tree of Knowledge. See the apples appearing on the Tree of Knowledge. See the serpent, the apples, and Eve all in the same instant.

BO3X - See and know the trees, the apples, Eve, and the serpent all in the same instant.

BO3X ▶ Know why even though God sent the serpent to test Adam and Eve, he still has to be punished.

BO3X ▶ See yourself as Eve leading Adam into life.

BO1X ▶ Know that by Adam's accepting to follow Eve, love can replace discord only by men accepting the wisdom of women.

CAIN AND ABEL: YOUR NATURE

BO3X ▶ Be Cain.

BO1X ▶ Be Abel. Who do you experience more strongly? Do not judge either.

BO3X ▶ As Abel, offer your first fruits to God. Know why you become closer to Him by this offering.

BO3X ▶ Know how we let the weak rule the strong in our everyday life.

BO1X ▶ Refuse to be sacrificed in this way.

BO3X ▶ Be your brother's keeper. What do you feel?

BO3X ▶ Feel and know how this quality brings peace and harmony to life.

BO2X ▶ Be Cain, wandering in the world with the mark on your forehead. Know what it is to wander in this way and why vengeance cannot be taken against you.

BO2X ▶ See, feel, and live as Cain, becoming the richest person in the world even though you have committed an iniquity. Know now how the quote "triumph of materialism" has brought decay to our lives individually and socially.

ABRAHAM: TO BECOME FAITHFUL

BO3X ▸ Hear as Abraham the command "Lech lecha" [from the Hebrew] "Go to yourself." Feel awakened, renewed, and resurrected.

BO3X ▸ Be as Abraham, the one of unsurpassed challenges, and feel the necessity to do them.

BO3X ▸ Live as Abraham the breaking of the idols.

BO3X ▸ Feel and know in yourself the total change and newness when breaking with the commonly accepted way to live.

BO3X ▸ Know and sense how all that has potential is now reality and is already present in you, always in you.

BO1X ▸ See and choose your own way. Have a blueprint of it and go ahead.

....

LOT AND LOT'S WIFE: TO EXPERIENCE RIGHTEOUSNESS AND EXPEL REGRET

BO3X ▸ See, sense, and feel yourself as Lot, righteous, generous, and understanding.

BO3X ▸ See and know the errors created by the men and women in Sodom and Gomorrah.

BO1X ▸ Now become aware of the errors you create in everyday life that create your own Sodom and Gomorrah, when you are not righteous, generous, and understanding.

BO3X ▸ Sense and feel the reluctance to leave people you love when it is necessary for you to take on a new way of life. Sense a moment of sadness at having no choice but to leave them.

BO1X ▸ Rejoice at the new choice you have made to turn to Spirit as your choice and theirs.

BO3X ▸ Become Lot's wife feeling regret at having to give up what is familiar. Sense this attachment to the past even though the past was or may have been painful. Sense and experience the tears welling up at seeing the loss associated with the past.

BO1X ▸ As the tears fall, see yourself becoming a pillar of salt, yourself hardening from the salt of the tears of regret about the past. Know how we become hardened when we attach ourselves to the pain of the past and the regrets connected with it.

BO2X ▸ Realize how all of these tears made you live disconnected from the present moment where all of our possibilities lie.

BO1X ▸ With a large hose of warm spiraling blue water, wash away all the salt from your body, inside and out. Feel yourself becoming renewed and revived with this newly found wisdom. Find yourself turned toward a new future and see what is there for you in this new instant.

JACOB: TO KNOW SELF-TRANSFORMATION

BO3X ▸ Be Jacob, the youth of contemplation.

BO1X ▸ Be Esau, the youth of cunning and hunting.

BO1X ▸ Choose who you wish to become. Do not judge your choice.

BO3X ▸ Go to Isaac as Jacob impersonating Esau. What do you feel? Hear what Isaac tells you and know your life's mission.

BO3X ▸ Work like Jacob for 14 years to fulfill your quest for what or whom you love. How do you feel? Know the true value of work.

BO2X ▸ Live and know Rebecca's deception against Esau.

BO2X ▸ Live and know Leah's deception against Jacob.

BO2X ▸ Live and know the deception of Jacob's sons falsely disclosing to Jacob that Joseph was dead.

BO3X ▸ Live, know, and feel without judgment the value of vice and deception.

BO3X ▸ Experience the ascending and descending of the angels on the ladder. See and feel the transformation coming with the presence of the ladder.

BO3X ▸ Let the angels escort you up the ladder. Be thankful for their presence.

BO2X ▸ Be as Jacob wrestling with the angel. Experience the struggle with God's messenger. Be grateful for the injury you sustain, reminding you of your spiritual transformation.

BO1X ▸ Hear your name being changed as the sound of this new name emanates. Know that your transformation is now in place.

JOSEPH: TO BECOME AWAKENED

BO3X ▸ Be as Joseph wearing your clean coat of many colors, telling your brothers the dream of the eleven sheaves of wheat. What do you experience through your senses and feelings?

BO1X ▸ Now see any of the brothers hearing the dream. What do you sense and feel?

BO1X ▸ See, sense, feel, and know yourself thrown in the pit. Understand why this was done to you. Let it now become a teacher to you.

BO3X ▸ With this new understanding, accept this new way of life away from everything familiar to you.

BO1X ▸ Know what it is to be "a stranger in a strange land."

BO3X ▸ Find yourself transformed into the master statesman, having used your gifts for the good of all. Know how using your gifts in this way made your transformation possible.

MOSES: TO BECOME A LEADER

BO3X ▸ See and feel yourself as Moses going up the mountainside with a flock of sheep. You come to the top and the sheep are grazing. Suddenly you feel intense heat all around you, enveloping you. Fire breaks out as the burning bush appears in front of you, cutting you off from the flock. What happens?

BO3X ▸ You are Moses, the Prince of Egypt. You are helping the Jews construct the pyramid. What happens?

BO3X ▸ You are Moses leading the people into the desert. Many of them are being bitten and poisoned by snakes. How do you feel and what do you do?

BO3X ▸ You are Moses climbing Mt. Sinai feeling yourself leaving the mass of people below. Finally, reaching the top, you sit and fast, asking God whatever question you wish answered. Then, with the tablets, descend the mountain and describe what happens.

BO3X ▸ You are Moses in the desert with the people. There is no water and the people are desperate for water. Experience the feelings of the people and the 70 elders. What do you find and what do you do?

BO3X ▸ The red heifer is in the desert. The specialists are showing the people the meaning of this cow. What is happening? Be among the people with the specialist and know the meaning of this cow.

....

INTENTION TO FIND SPIRITUAL FREEDOM

BO3X ▸ Live and know how freedom can be connected directly to our physical relationship to life.

BO3X ▸ See, feel, and sense why without being in a physical body, freedom cannot happen.

BO1X ▸ Experience yourself as a dot in the center of a circle.

BO1X ▸ See, sense, and live the present moment as no time.

BO3X ▸ Sense and feel how the imagery process allows us to live the presence of the present.

Seeking Truth The Christian Way

"I live in time and out of time, by inner experience. For all of us, at every instant it is possible to do so, if, only, quiet and calm, we live with the moment... But the key is in living fully. Bringing every instant To its eternity."
-Colette, "How to Live"

THE PRAYER OF SAINT FRANCIS

BO3X ▸ See, feel, and know, "Lord, make me an instrument of your peace."

BO1X ▸ "Lord, where there is hatred, let there be love."

BO1X ▸ "Lord, where there is injury, let me bring pardon."

BO3X ▸ "Lord, where there is doubt, let me bring faith."

BO1X ▸ "Lord, where there is despair, let me bring hope."

BO1X ▸ "Lord, where there is sadness, let me bring joy."

BO1X ▸ "Lord, where there is darkness, let me bring light."

BO3X ▸ There is a seal that is not engraved. Engrave on it an image or work of what you want to become.

BO1X ▸ Now engrave this on your heart and feel what happens.

....

ROAD TO SPIRIT: TIME ▸ FROM *HEBREW THOUGHT COMPARED WITH GREEK*: BY THORLIEF BOMAN

BO3X ▸ See, live, and feel the difference between complete and past.

BO3X ▸ Know and live how time is determined by its content.

BO1X ► See and know that time is occurrence and stream of events.

BO3X ► Know and live that time is intensity.

BO3X ► See and feel the difference between time-rhythm and time-movement.

BO3X ► See and know the difference between contemporaneous (happening during the same period of time) and modern (recent time or present).

BO1X ► Now become contemporaneous with Abraham.

BO1X ► Now become contemporaneous with Moses.

BO1X ► Now become contemporaneous with Buddha.

BO1X ► Now become contemporaneous with Jesus.

BO1X ► Now become contemporaneous with Mohammed.

....

THE THREE VOWS: OBEDIENCE

BO3X ► See, feel, sense, know, and live the prayer, "Hear, Oh Israel, the Lord is your God. The Lord is One. Blessed be His name forever and ever."

BO3X ► Feel, live, and know the command, "Love God with all your heart, all your soul, and all your might."

BO3X ▸ Hear your name being called from Above. Answer, "Here I am Lord." What do you feel?

....

THE THREE VOWS: CHASTITY

BO3X ▸ Feel and know the meaning of the biblical comment, "Thou shall have no other gods before me."

BO3X ▸ See and sense yourself separating the wheat from the chaff.

BO1X ▸ See the golden grains of wheat filter through your fingers until one grain remains in your palm.

BO1X ▸ See this grain become the sun in the seed sending golden light to illumine your heart.

BO3X ▸ See yourself in the mirror naked. In this instant see and clean any blemishes and impurities.

BO1X ▸ Turn over the mirror. See your new pure self. Wipe the image away to the right with your right hand.

....

THE THREE VOWS: POVERTY

BO3X ▸ Imagine yourself in the room most important or significant to you now or in your childhood. Starting from the door, look into the room at everything from the left to the right. Clear the room from the top down, starting with the ceiling and walls and going down to the floor. Remove all the articles on the ceiling and walls and bring them to the center of the room.

BO1X ▸ Furnish all the necessary implements, including a ladder, to clean the high places. Clean the room in general. As you work your way to the floor level, bring all articles to the center of the room. Take the books from the bookcases and other areas of the room and place them in the center of the room.

BO1X ▸ Place a container, such as a trunk or box, in the center of the room to hold all the articles you will discard. After everything is in the center of the room, place it in the container, noticing what you are discarding. Take the container out through the doorway.

Wash all the windows from top to bottom, left to right. After rolling up the carpet and placing it in the center of the room, clean the floor. If you wish to dust or polish the furniture, do so.

BO1X ▸ Now take the container of discards to a large field and burn it, watching the flames. If the container is metal, see it sinking in the ocean and watch the eddies as it sinks and disappears. Be aware of your thoughts and feelings when watching the container burn or sink.

BO1X ▸ Come back into the room. See it anew, noting any feeling and remembering them.

Clarity

"My knowledge comes from my Images.
I sense, hear, See. And I know why verity becomes Beauty
And is adorning us with the white mantle of clarity."
-Colette, "The White Mantle"

BECOMING CLEAR AND TRANSPARENT: FOR DETOXIFICATION

BO3X ▸ See and feel the psychic winds as blue light, sounding sweetly.

BO1X ▸ Sense it entering your body, slowly feeling it.

BO1X ▸ See and sense your body filled with blue light.

BO3X ▸ See and hear the blue psychic wind cleaning out of the body all that has to be cleansed, by dissolving it.

BO1X ▸ Feel and see your solar plexus as a knot, untied and unraveled by the process of fulfillment of the blue light.

BLUE MEADOW

BO3X ▸ Enter the blue meadow. Everything is blue, the grass, trees, flowers—everything is blue. There are many pools or lakes in this meadow.

BO1X ▸ Enter the pool for frustration. Immerse yourself fully, cleansing yourself thoroughly of that feeling.

BO1X ▸ Jump across an open part of the meadow into the pool for resentment. Immerse yourself fully, cleansing yourself thoroughly of that feeling.

BO1X ▸ Jump across an open part of the meadow into the pool for anger. Immerse yourself fully, cleansing yourself thoroughly of that feeling.

BO1X ▸ Jump across an open part of the meadow into the pool for regret. Immerse yourself fully, cleansing yourself thoroughly of that feeling.

BO1X ▸ Jump across an open part of the meadow into the pool for guilt, immersing three times, cleansing yourself fully of that feeling.

BO1X ► Jump across an open part of the meadow into the pool of well-being. Come out and lie down in the meadow covering yourself with the light coming from the blue flowers surrounding and penetrating you.

BO3X ► From the hollow parts of your body sense your energy and gather your breathing.

BO1X ► Move it with your hands. Envelop it with your arms.

BO1X ► Be aware of the movement of your breathing until not feeling and sensing it.

BO1X • Sense the breath disappearing and transforming in the instant into the power of Spirit. Sense this in your hands.

SEEING INSIDE ONESELF

BO3X ► It is evening with a full moon reflecting in a clear pool of water. Looking into the pool, see the reflection of the moon. See your face in the crystal pool.

BO1X ► Move now further to the left and look at your reflected face in the silvery light of the moon.

BO1X ► Go to a place between these reflective faces and see your face once again. Make any changes you want to in your face, if you are not satisfied with it.

THE TOWER: THE BEST

BO3X ► You are in the top of a tower waiting for the best to come. It is coming toward you. Step out of the tower and take a step above it, seeing all around you and then seeing the best coming toward you.

WEIGHTS

BO3X ► Have your arms hanging at your side and feel your hands weighted down by hundreds of pounds of weights on each. Feel heaviness ascending up your arms, then descending down the spinal column to the coccyx. Sense your body lengthening. Feel the coccyx and sense the heaviness ascending up from the floor of the pelvis, the lower abdomen, upper abdomen, chest, and mouth into the nose.

BO3X ▸ Sense your breathing in your nose and mouth.

BO3X ▸ Sense your breathing in all of your organs and then having perfect emptiness. See yourself filling your organs by keeping in yourself integrity and spontaneity.

BO1X ▸ See your body as a crystal vase filled with blue water.

BO3X ▸ Sense and feel that another universe is filling the center of your body in the core of the core.

FROM *TRAVEL DIARIES OF A PHILOSOPHER:* BY COUNT HERMANN KEYSERLING*

BO3X ▸ Ask God to bring you from non-reality to reality.

BO3X ▸ Ask God to bring you from darkness to light.

BO3X ▸ Ask God to bring us from death, bringing us to immortality.

BO1X ▸ Become what you are!

BO3X ▸ Displace the order of nature. Go in the opposite direction and reach The Source.

TO CROSS A BRIDGE BACKWARDS

BO3X ▸ See yourself as a being of sand. Be all the sensations and feelings.

BO3X ▸ See that you want to break with a part of the past but the man or woman of sand in you has not the courage to take the decision.

BO1X ▸ See how you have decided to cross the bridge, but as it is difficult to cut briskly with the past, you try to cross the bridge backward.

BO3X ▸ Say something nice to people you love as you cross this bridge backwards. When you are at the beginning of the bridge look at all the beings who stay behind. Remember the links you have had with them. Send each of them a nice thought. Ignore the ones who have hurt or harmed you.

BO1X ▸ See how you are crossing the bridge backwards slowly, trying to keep your balance and your pace and seeing friends and family diminishing in size.

BO1X ▸ See how you are reaching the end of the bridge. Send a last look to your past. Know it is the last look.

BO1X ▸ See how you are putting a bomb at your feet, adding the string or fuse and lighting it. Turning around, walk away without turning your head, without knowing what has happened.

BO1X ▸ See how in doing so, you have increased your strength and accepted the uncertainty.

CLEANSING FOR RENEWAL

BO3X ▸ With a candle in your hand, enter a room. With the light of the candle, look at what is hidden and waiting for you in the four corners of the room.

BO1X ▸ Going to the first corner in front of you, see what is there.

BO1X ▸ Walking to the right, bring your light into the next corner.

BO1X ▸ Walking to the right, go to the third corner and have the light of your candle discovering what is there.

BO1X ▸ Go to the fourth corner and look at it clearly to find what is there for you.

BO3X ▸ Know that you have to sacrifice everything to the truth you are discovering.

IMMOBILITY OR ELIXIR OF LIFE:
FOR BACK TROUBLES

BO3X ► Imagine yourself in a posture.

BO1X ► Sense and feel the physical and psychological benefit of keeping your posture. Sense the effect of immobility in combination with relaxation.

BO3X ► Sense how the lowering of metabolic levels of the body is reducing stress by slowing and quieting.

BO3X ► Sense how refraining from movements also has strengthening effects, brings self-confidence, and allows the expressing of will.

BO3X ► Live and know how suppression of movement has a liberating effect on the mind.

BO3X ► Feel and know how accepting the leg pain coming from long-sitting meditation asks for courage and brings self-respect.

BO1X ► Know how this courage and self-respect are taking us away from anomie, a sickness of the soul in which you are experiencing no meaning in life.

BO3X ► Feel and know how the attitude of the hero is the real elixir of life.

....

FOR BRAIN BALANCE

BO3X ► Into a mirror see yourself becoming immobile like a mummy.

BO1X ► See how the aorta is beating more and more slowly. Sense it until a special frequency follows its beat, traveling through the body and reverberating in the third ventricle* of the brain.

BO1X ► Sense how the wave that is set up is traveling in the sensory motor area, ending in the pleasure center of the hypothalamus.

TREE EXERCISE: FOR HEALING CANCER

BO3X ▸ See and feel how you are like a tree planted by the stream of water.

BO1X ▸ See and feel how you are bringing forth your fruit in the season.

BO1X ▸ Feel and see how your leaves do not wither.

BO1X ▸ Feel and see how in all you do, you will prosper.

ORANGE: FOR PAIN RELIEF

BO3X ▸ See an orange and slice it. Put a slice onto the pained area and know that slice is absorbing the pain. Now put the slice back into the orange, as you put the orange back together.

LIVE YOUR BODY AND YOUR BODY LIVES: TO MAINTAIN HEALTH

BO3X ▸ Sense and recognize how we are going out of the center as a way to find more acceptable outside ways.

BO3X ▸ Feel how when not to go out of ourselves we have to find new ways of enjoyment and truth.

BO1X ▸ See how we have to return to ourselves to recognize the inside joy and its roots.

BO3X ▸ See and know how all asceticism is constructed on the initial joy coming from your body.

BO1X ▸ Feel and know how by stopping this joy, we find a higher level of joy that is permitting us to leap to Spirit.

BO3X ▸ Live, sense, and know how living the body from the outside is causing you to have stored memories and blocked emotions.

BO3X ▸ Live and know how finding your body for itself in its specificity is happening only from the inside.

BO3X ▸ Know and live how more of being is coming to you when the form of emptiness is filled.

BO1X ▸ Feel this filled form pushing you outside.

BO3X ▸ Live how stress coming from lack becomes obsessive when well-being cannot be reached.

BO1X ▸ And refuse this obsessive way. What do you experience?

Transforming The Evil Impulse

"Evil is only part of the whole,
And Cain, brother of the good."
-Colette, "Bi-Reality"

GOING FROM DARK TO LIGHT:
FOR MENTAL AND EMOTIONAL HEALTH

BO3X ▸ See the inherited and inherent power in yourself and the power that each person you meet gives you.

BO3X ▸ See how when using Imagery for an acute or chronic problem, well-chosen images are promoting the potential for ordering the disorder.

BO3X ▸ See how with Imagery you are finding your natural state of health.

BO3X ▸ See how in happiness, fulfillment, and love you are making every moment with Imagery a moment of wondrous creation in which we naturally choose the best.

BO3X ▸ Imagine yourself smiling freely and sense how you relax.

BO1X ▸ See how this facilitates states of mind beneficial to effect change.

BO3X ▸ See how you are creating the clear idea of what is desired and the possibility or possibilities of obtaining it.

BO3X ▸ Live, see, and feel that in our minds what feels sometimes as dangerous, evil, or non-healthy is the source of richness and how we have to control them by prudence, measure, and self-observation.

BO3X ▸ Live, feel, and see your own recovered psychic health flourishing by a higher self control.

BO1X • Live, feel, and see your own recovered psychic health flourishing as non-repressive.

BO1X ► Live, feel, and see your own recovered psychic health flourishing productively.

BO3X ► Live, feel, and see your own recovered psychic health flourishing in spontaneity.

BO1X ► Live, feel, and see your own recovered psychic health flourishing as authenticity.

BO1X ► Live, feel, and see your own recovered psychic health flourishing as self-accomplishment.

BO3X ► Live, feel, and see your own recovered psychic health flourishing in maturity.

BO1X ► Live, feel, and see your own recovered psychic health flourishing as self-realization.

BO1X ► Live, feel, and see your own recovered psychic health flourishing in plenitude.

BO3X ► Sense how by Imagery we recognize illness as a message from within.

BO1X ► Know how by using images you unmask the meaning of disease and transform the dysfunction into an enriching experience for yourself.

BO3X ► See how Imagery gives you the opportunity to develop intuition, inventiveness and to promote curing and creativity.

BO3X ► See how Imagery gives you the opportunity to extend this understanding of the interplay of the organism with the surrounding environment.

BO3X ► Sense and feel how Imagery is one of the main tools to improve learning, stop resistance and may be seen as a vital factor for correcting any form of dysfunction or disease.

BO3X ▸ See how images are the bridge for harmony, meaning, and healing.

BO3X ▸ See images as a privileged discipline to improve lifestyle, for helping people, or to live as long as possible.

FOR HEALING

BO3X ▸ Sense the anguish coming from an agonizing physical pain.

BO1X ▸ Sense how angst is provoking a constriction, narrowness, and physical sensation of being tied up.

BO3X ▸ Feel how nameless disturbing or distressing sensations are causing an anxiety that is in apprehension, bringing torment that makes you emotionally ill.

BO3X ▸ Sense your throat or your heart or your solar plexus or your stomach tied up by a rope with a strong knot. Undo the knot every morning when you get up. What do you sense and feel?

BO3X ▸ Sense that when you embrace the one you love, they may sense that as being squeezed or strangled.

BO1X ▸ Know how an intensity may bring to the other angst, anguish, and anxiety.

INTO THE NIGHT OF THE SOUL:
BY VARIOUS AFRICAN POETS

BO3X ▸ Hear the sound in your blood and feel all this life in your blood.

BO3X ▸ Hear the song that is whipping your blood.

BO3X ▸ Recognize and remember the rhythm that is hunting away anxiety.

BO3X ▸ Listen to the voice of water, the water that is speaking.

BO1X ▸ See the earth listening to the voice of water.

BO1X ▸ See the fire listening to the voice of water, this water that is listened to.

BO1X ▸ This fire that tells the wind where it has to go.

BO3X ▸ Listen to the wind that brings the bush into movement.

BO1X ▸ Listen to this bush where you sweetly hear the soul of nature.

Awareness

"…But, experiencing, I have seen that mind is changing the world, and changing you, and me."
-Colette, "Eating the Menu Instead of the Meal"

FIRST FRUITS: FROM RABBI NACHMAN

BO3X ▸ See, sense, feel, live, and know the statement of his, "Master of the Universe, awesome and dreadful, give me the new words right now. Give me just now the right words able to make us calm, peaceful and true here and now, that permit me with joy to return in truth to You just now."

FROM THE PROPHET AMOS

BO3X ▸ See, feel, and know justice rushing at us as waves of truth, as an eternal torrent, returning you to yourself.

BO3X ▸ Sense at what point to use your human knowledge and influence to activate the one channel you have chosen to work with.

BO1X ▸ Sense and know how by means of that influx you may create in the image of God whatever you feel is right to create.

BO1X ▸ Know how if your wish is selfish, you are no more in the image of God and become powerless forever.

VOLUNTARY SIMPLICITY AS A STATE OF BEING

BO3X ▸ Feel and know voluntary simplicity as a bridge making a transition between worlds.

BO1X ▸ Feel and know that voluntary simplicity, being a state of being, is a new frontier.

BO3X ▸ See and know how and where your life is unnecessarily complicated.

BO3X ▸ Feel and see how you are aware of the distractions, clutter, and pretense that inform your life.

BO3X ▸ See and know how our pretense makes passage through the world cumbersome and awkward.

BO1X ▸ See and live how true voluntary simplicity makes us live clearly and lightly.

BO3X ▸ Know and understand how that which you have imagined contributes to the emerging global sense of reality that embraces human unity and diversity.

BO3X ▸ See and understand how human beings are not separate atoms, and serve their unity.

BO3X ▸ See and know why the meeting of West and East is succeeding now because the world mastery of the West and the self-mastery of the East are putting the future in our hands.

....

STATES OF BEING

BO3X ▸ Feel and know how without fear and anxiety we may reach the other states of being that are within us.

BO3X ▸ See and know how the modern answer to suffering is work, which brings an income, ability to relax, retreat, the possibility of retirement, medical support, and some leisure.

BO3X ▸ See and live how this work, when not completely accepted, is imprisonment and when not accepted with love is sleep.

BO3X ▸ Feel and know that regardless of your actual age and success, this real waking life promises the fulfillment of being.

BO4X ▸ Know and feel how it is difficult to be different and how you are when people see you differently.

BO3X ▸ Know that to seek different states of being asks for:

BO1X ▸ Courage

BO1X ▸ Constancy

BO1X ▸ Determination

BO3X ▸ Know and feel how because body and skin is the way we relate to others, reaching transcendental states demands that we change the working of the body.

....

ISIS, ARCHETYPAL JOURNEY ▸ WISDOM OF PAST AND FUTURE EXPERIENCED IN THE MOMENT: FOR CREATIVITY AND TRANSFORMATION

BO4X ▸ Feel and see yourself as the Goddess Isis re-assembling the dismembered body of Osiris.

BO1X ▸ See yourself as Isis re-membering him.

BO3X ▸ Feel and know how remembrance is putting in at the right place and at the right time the different parts to make with them a living whole.

BO3X ▸ See, know, and feel how remembering is a restorative and creative act.

BO2X ▸ See and know how by remembering, we recreate someone by taking bits of scattered facts and recreating his or her image.

BO3X ▸ See and feel how to recreate this image, you have to add an important part of yourself so that you are creating a new entity.

BO3X ▸ Know and feel how by remembering, you are bringing the forgotten one back to a new wholeness and by reinstalling him or her in the external world, you bring him or her into existence.

BO3X ▸ Feel and know how by immersing himself into the depths of a deep woman, man comes to know himself.

BO3X ▸ See and feel how by looking into the image of the deep unconsciousness, we come to know ourselves.

BO3X ▸ See yourself breathing out gray smoke and breathing in blue light. Feel and know that a real woman is the vessel of transformation and transposition and why the seekers after The Grail vessel had at first to find the right woman.

BO3X ▸ See and live how winged inspiration has to be caught, brought back to earth, and grounded in reality. If not, it scatters itself aimlessly.

BO3X ▸ See and live how it is through highly spiritualized women like Isis, that Spirit, coming out of nature and having broken with nature, is recaptured, realized, and brought down to reality.

BO3X ▸ See, live, and know why at the base of the Isis statue in Egypt is written, "I am everything that was, that is, that ever will be. Nor has any mortal man ever to discover what lies under my veil."

Plotinus*

"...the key is in living fully.
Bringing every instant to its eternity."
-Colette, "How to Live"

WELL-BEING: FOR BECOMING WHOLE, HEALTHY, AND HOLY

Let your mind and heart release all that disturbs you. Let your body, all its frets and all that surrounds it be still. Let the earth and sea and air be still and heaven itself. And then think of Spirit as streaming, pouring, rushing, and shining into you, through you and out from you in all directions while you sit quietly.

BO3X ▸ See and sense how well-being is a normal part of life.

BO1X ▸ See, sense, and feel how well-being is living well.

BO1X ▸ See, sense, and feel how living well-being is the superabundance of life.

BO1X ▸ See, sense, and feel how a superabundant life is the "best" and makes you really alive and you then have a perfect life.

BO3X ▸ Sense, feel, and know how true life is the Transcendent Intelligible Reality.

BO1X ▸ Know how we are in the image or trace of that Intelligible Reality.

BO1X ▸ Know how this experience cannot be gained from any source outside ourselves.

BO3X ▸ See, sense, feel, and live how identity with the Transcendent Good is perfect life.

BO1X ▸ See and know how living the virtuous life is our way as humans to identify with the Transcendent Good.

BO3X ▸ See, sense, and know how to have the life of the Transcendent Good is to have all we need.

BO1X ▸ See and sense how to have a virtuous life is all that is needed for well-being and the acquisition of the good.

BO3X ▸ Feel and know that by living the virtuous life, we give the body what it needs without taking anything away from our own life.

BO3X ▸ See, live, and know how even when fortune goes against you, the good life is still there.

BO3X ▸ See, sense, feel, live, and know how by living in virtue you know what death really is for you and that of your friends and relations.

BO1X ▸ Know how with this knowledge and understanding, death of others causes grief, but doesn't grieve you.

BO3X ▸ See and know how the good man will not be involved in evil because of the stupidity of others, even if they are his relatives.

BO1X ▸ See and know how he will not be dependent on the good or bad fortune of other people.

BO3X ▸ See and know how for the good man, none of his experiences penetrate to the inner self, neither pleasures nor pains, any more than others.

BO3X ▸ Do not behave like someone untrained, but stand up to the blows of life like a trained fighter. Know that your own nature can bear them, not as terrors, but as children's bogeymen.

BO1X ▸ Know how the man of well-being sets virtue and good against misfortune, making his soul hard to disturb or distress.

BO3X ▸ See, sense, feel, live, and know how the good man is always happy, his state is tranquil, his disposition contented and undisturbed by any so-called evils.

BO1X ▸ Sense and know how if everyone looks for another kind of pleasure in the life of virtue, it is not the life of virtue he is looking for.

BO3X ▸ See, know, and live how a good man's activities are not hindered by change of fortune, but adapt to circumstances.

BO3X ► See, sense, feel, live, and know how well-being is not determined by the state of the body, not by its size, health, excellence of its senses, nor by being in a state of pain or pleasure.

BO1X ► Realize that nothing can add to or diminish your state of well-being.

BO3X ► See, feel, and know how well-being comes from there and not from here.

BO3X ► Sense and feel how you give to your bodily life as much as it needs, but you are other than it and can abandon it.

BO3X ► See, sense, and know how you do not call things terrible or frightening, but have the confidence that evil cannot touch you.

BO3X ► Live and know how well-being is living in eternity not in time and that the passage of time cannot affect it.

BO3X ► See, feel, and live how your inner state produces well-being and it does not come from something outside of yourself.

BO1X ► Know how virtue resides inwardly.

BO3X ► See, feel, and know how memory plays no part in well-being nor is well-being a matter of talking.

BO1X ► Feel and know how well-being is being in a particular state. A state is something present and so is an actuality of life.

BO3X ► Know it is not correct to count your pleasures in reckoning well-being. Know that well-being has a boundary and a limit and is always the same.

BO3X ► "Measure well-being by the present and you make it indivisible. Deepen the present moment and you have the 'Image of Eternity.'" – Plotinus

BO3X ▸ See, sense, feel, live, and know how well-being is not counted by time, but by eternity.

BO1X ▸ See, feel, and know how it is not measured by extension but by "This here — un-extended and timeless."

BO3X ▸ Sense and know how eternity is from the whole of time: It is not made up of many times.

BO3X ▸ See, feel, and sense how well-being is not increased by time nor by numbers of actions, for a non-active person can be in well-being.

BO1X ▸ See and live how well-being is an inner state unrelated to external actions and is therefore unaffected by time.

Regaining Health and Wholeness: To Your Health

"In us, the Tree of Life ever new, ever green,
Is crowned by the conjunction of the two blue stars.
They unify the core of the living body…"
-Colette, "The Blue Stars Conjunction"

DISCIPLINE

BO3X ► Imagine how in modern education as well as in self-education we are valuing spontaneity and letting go.

BO3X ► Sense what is inherently healthy in accepting discipline and pursuing a disciplined life.

BO3X ► Live and know how to organize your own day around what has value and meaning for yourself. Sense its worth.

BO1X ► See and live how when the day-to-day decisions and activities have been organized and accepted, your attention is freed for inside work.

BO3X ► See and know how it is possible to accept a task from a teacher, a master, a cleric.

BO3X ► Sense how the feeling that is coming from this freely accepted task is permitting you progress, development, and some cures.

BO3X ► See and live how the example and teaching of a master teacher and disciple is bringing new energy and a new future.

BO3X ► Sense how some major life changes may happen.

BO3X ▸ Live how some destructive habit has been abandoned under the direction of a good teacher and a good example.

BO3X ▸ Live how you are minimizing stress by regulating normal function: food intake, sleep, activity, sexual activity. Sense this pressure being reduced.

BO3X ▸ Live how by synchronizing your body clock daily, you are improving physical and emotional functioning.

BO3X ▸ See yourself inside a cube.

BO1X ▸ See yourself in a sphere within a cube. If constricted, change the limits of the sphere.

BO1X ▸ And feel yourself calm now.

BEING PLAYED UPON

BO3X ▸ Looking into a mirror or screen, see and live how we are born on a stage in the middle of a play we did not write.

BO3X ▸ Feel, live, and know to what extent can we act here in life and on the stage.

BO1X ▸ Live and know whether we are playing the parts assigned to us or are the parts playing us.

BO3X ▸ See and feel if we are tricked or falling into our own trap.

BO1X ▸ Live how we are fooled by ourselves as long as we believe we are being those characters we are playing.

PLAYED BY OUR OWN ROLES

BO3X ► Live and know how we are played by our own roles as long as they are more real for us than our unseen reality.

BO3X ► See and live how when looking at a costumed and masked character, it seems that we confuse what we see with the being behind them.

BO1X ► See how we are taking the role for the player.

BO3X ► See how we know that an actor, playing Hamlet, is never Hamlet. We do not expect this of him.

BO3X - Now live how we expect our father to be The Father, reducing The Father to our father's performance.

BO1X ► See how when we are the father or mother, we reduce The Father and The Mother to ourselves.

TO REACH THE GOAL

BO3X ► See the one task you have to achieve.

BO1X ► See it in all the details of its development.

BO1X ► See it completely achieved and successful.

BO1X ► See the best results for the country and the world.

BO3X ► See and feel how the Absolute Mind (God) seems to help your mind conceive the perfect task for the perfect result.

BO1X ► See that when you have forgotten yourself, it has directed all of you in the right way.

BO3X ► Know that when your mind is connected with the Absolute Mind, the right image will immediately bring the desired effect in our lower world.

BO3X ► Know that all you have learned to be nearer The Absolute now has its reward, permitting you to act for the good of the country, the world, and yourself.

BO3X ► Know that when the intention of your prayer is for a non-egoistic purpose, there is no barrier between your praying and a reaction to your prayer.

BO3X ► Sense how the vibrations you are emitting are reaching the All Knowing Mind and are making your intention actual in the instant.

BO3X ► Feel and see how your own vibrations are connected with the vibration of the All Knowing Mind and sense how the entire cosmos is vibrating in response to your prayer.

BO3X ► See how by the intention of your prayer coming into action you are ready for The Receiving and The Union.

LAYING-ON THE HANDS

BO3X ► Imagine that you lie down attuned to your own sensations and feelings.

BO1X ► Imagine rubbing your hands together. Have them face each other.

BO1X ► Imagine placing your hands on your pelvic bones.

BO1X ► Imagine focusing your awareness between the exchange between hands and bones.

BO3X ► Release this awareness and feel yourself being held.

BO1X ► What is occurring in your body (sensations, body emanations, dream images, good, and forgotten memories)?

BO3X ► Imagine placing your hands at your sides.

BO1X ► Feel and know how your body feels differently.

BO1X ► Imagine coming slowly to one inch of your body and move your hands all along it. Trust your hands. Feel the emanations of your body from neck to toes and hands.

BO1X ► Sense the places that feel stronger or weaker, congested, depleted, or numb. Massage with a circular motion any area of tension.

BO3X ► Imagine allowing your hands to make full contact and be totally aware of your position.

The Healthy Ways

"Health, as joyful fullness, has never been our every day reward. But if it happens, in happiness, we live the glorious richness of Triumphant Epiphany, in us, the Tree of Life ever new, ever green…"
-Colette, "The Blue Stars Conjunction"

GREEN THUMB

BO3X ▸ Imagine that you have a green thumb.

BO1X ▸ See and live how with your green thumb you are growing up healthy.

BO3X ▸ Imagine that you have a green thumb.

BO1X ▸ See and live how with your green thumb you are making some chosen others grow up healthy.

BO3X ▸ Imagine that you have a green thumb.

BO1X ▸ See and live how you are now making all the human beings in the world grow up healthy. What is happening?

THE BEGINNING OF LIGHT OR WHAT IS NOT YET HEARD

BO3X ▸ See and live the uncreated light of The Beginning and of The End.

BO1X ▸ See and sense yourself attracted by the vibration of this light. Feel being taken into the light by the vibration of the tremendous sound coming out of The Beginning and The End.

BO1X ▸ See and sense how returning from the light and sound, we have returned to ourselves and are no more in exile on the earth.

BO3X ▸ See and sense how like Abraham you are able to sacrifice the credibility and possibility of the past in its own richness and beauty for the truth of now.

BO3X ▸ Feel and see how by that sacrifice you are reintegrating the Evident Ultimate Light.

DAWN WELCOMES OUR DEEP STARRY NIGHT

BO3X ▸ Look at the starry night. Try to recognize stars and constellations.

BO1X ▸ Imagine Orion upside down becoming the Southern Cross.

BO1X ▸ See and know that a different point of view is provoking a great reversing.

BO3X ▸ Look at a new dawn and let its dim light become the starry black velvet of the night.

BO3X ▸ Bending in front of Orion and the Southern Cross, feel and sense the wind of dawn and hear it around and in you.

BO1X ▸ Sense the might and power of the instant of separation between night and day.

BO!X – Feel and recognize the sacredness of the moment.

BO1X ▸ Hear what the wind of dawn is telling you.

THE THROAT

BO3X ▸ Sense and see your throat as the crossing point and the point of reversing everything in our being.

BO1X ▸ Sense and see your throat as the crossing point and the point of reversing of the emotional center of the solar plexus.

BO1X ▸ Sense and see your throat as the crossing point and the point of reversing of the sensitivity center of the heart.

BO3X ▸ Imagine an overwhelming emotion. Sense and see how it is located in the solar plexus.

BO1X ▸ Sense how it is felt in the throat, where its intensity is reversed before reaching the brain.

BO3X ▸ Do the same with the deep feeling sensed in your heart, reversed in your throat before reaching the brain.

REDUCING STRESS
BASED ON FEAR OF AGGRESSION

BO3X - See and feel what is happening in yourself and others when you are distancing human aggression.

BO1X ▸ See and feel what is happening in yourself when you are tranquilizing human aggression.

BO1X ▸ See and feel what is happening in yourself when you are numbing human aggression.

BO3X ▸ See that if you succeed, the price is disinterest.

BO3X ▸ See and sense aggression as an effective force in shaping yourself and others' behavior.

BO1X ▸ See yourself learning and practicing different fight styles for minimizing hurtful hostility.

BO3X ▸ Use a fair fight and understand this exchange between you and a friend.

BO1X ▸ Use a fair fight and understand this exchange between you and a competitor.

BO1X • Use a fair fight and understand this exchange between you and a loved one. Sense this emotional interdependence.

BO3X ▸ Using a fair fight in your couple relationship, find how you are negotiating change. Sense the pleasure and even the joy that grows out of that. See how productive it is.

BO3X ► Find a personal way to change this aggression.

BO1X ► See how with this you have removed punishment, hurtful hostility, vengefulness, distrust, smarting, and irrational emotions.

BO1X ► Know that you are now realistic in your fair fight.

BO3X ► See yourself removing the escalating hostility of generalizations and rigid stereotypes.

BO3X ► See how this life, by these ways, brings you much information about options and non-negotiable territories.

BO3X ► Sense how this fair fight is a communication and training for dealing with one issue, a specific behavior pattern which carries with it a will for change.

....

FAIR FIGHT FOR CHANGE

BO3X ► Sense and see that you have to use conflicts and aggression creatively.

BO3X ► Feel how to stop the hostile hurt-oriented and harmful component of your aggression.

BO3X ► Into a screen see yourself as the "nice one" with an uncritical, unconditional, positive regard for the other. Then see three different people, one at home, one at work, one in larger society and apply "nice one."

BO3X ► See how this unconditional regard as the "nice one" doesn't help the others move to a constructive experience.

BO3X ► Into the mirror look now at yourself with a critical, aggressive, even a fighting confrontation with the same people.

BO3X ► See how when you do this without hate or revenge, you open these people to a new attitude that permits them to consider new alternative ways for solving conflicts.

BO3X ► Sense and feel that if threat is happening, then an open display of aggression may occur.

BO1X ► Sense and feel that if trust is happening, the open display of aggression may not occur.

BO3X ► See how trust is the shield that avoids hurtful hostility and facilitates good combatants to fight fairly.

BO1X ► See how this fair fight is not against each other, but is for improvement in this relationship.

MIRRORING TO SAY GOODBYE

BO3X ► Into the mirror see two memories of bad moments.

BO1X • Into the mirror see two memories of good moments.

BO1X ► Into the mirror see two dreams.

BO1X ► Into the mirror see the forever.

BO1X ► Into the mirror see your marriage or a close relationship.

BO1X ► Into the mirror see what you have learned and say goodbye to these memories.

THE COMPLETE EXERCISE

BO3X ► See yourself in a cave with paintings of ancient animals on the walls. These animals come alive.

BO1X ▸ You take your belt and lasso the one you are most afraid of. Ascend from the cave, taking the animal with you. See it in the light of day being desiccated by the sun. Bury what is left.

BO1X ▸ Ascend a staircase that is where you are. Going up five steps, remove your coat. Going up five steps, remove your shirt. Going up five steps, remove your shoes. Going up five steps, remove your socks. Going up five steps, remove your pants or skirt. Going up five steps, remove your underwear.

BO1X ▸ Climb 15 steps to the 45th step. Throw away anything you may be carrying. Here find yourself close to God and know that God is near you. See your nakedness, covered by a mantle of light. Descend more quickly to the base of the staircase. See the staircase becoming glistening white. Find the discarded clothes at the base. Bury them in a hole and cover them with earth. Put on your new everyday clothes still covered by the light. See the aura and its color, but not the halo and the head.

BO1X ▸ Return to your everyday life, sensing and feeling all that has gone on.

Images of The Heart:
For Repairing Heart Disorders

"I love and I am more, I love and I am not.
Where is it coming from, this ambiguous love?"
-Colette, "The Love of My Being"

TRAVEL OF THE HEART OF AN EMBRYO

BO3X ▸ Feel yourself as an embryo, small and floating in the womb.

BO1X ▸ Sense your heart on your right shoulder, then follow it moving along the new delicate bones of the top of the ribs along your trunk. It is a warm, glowing color.

BO1X ▸ Follow your heart around the ribs of the right side.

BO1X ▸ Sense the diaphragm sitting in the middle of the open body and becoming steady. You settle your heart in its just and comfortable place in coordination with the lungs and solar plexus.

BO1X ▸ Sense your heart traveling to take its right place and position above the diaphragm.

COEUR A COEUR

BO3X ▸ Sense and feel that your heart is concretely touching the heart of someone you love and is understanding you.

BO3X ▸ With elongated fingers and your hands full of light, enlarge the space around your heart and the other tissue nearby. Have this space full of light.

BO1X ▸ With your fingers open your heart. Look at the tree in your heart or breast or chest.

BO3X ▸ Go into your heart and into your hand that is in your tree. What is happening?

BO1X ► Go into your heart and into the tree that is in your heart. How are you living it?

BO1X ► Go into your heart and into the eye that is in your heart. How are you seeing? How are you feeling with the all-seeing eye? See your sensing and see your feelings.

BO1X ► Go into your heart and into the star that is now in your heart. What is happening?

BO3X ► Sense how the sound of the palpitations of the star and its vibrating light are curing all the malaise and difficulties of everyday life.

BO1X ► Sense and feel what is happening when the space is free in your heart.

BO3X ► Go into your heart and into the hand that is in your heart. What is happening?

BO3X ► See yourself jumping out of your heart, then go into your heart and be throwing your heart overhead and seeing the vibration and palpitation of light in your heart.

AGAINST THE HEART

BO1X ► Confront your heart. See yourself doing something important, going against this heart feeling.

GREEN LEAF TO RENEW AND REJUVENATE THE HEART

BO3X ▸ Have a rake and leaf broom. Be in a garden in the Fall. Rake the leaves and sweep them to the corner of the garden in a pile ready for removal. Burn them and bury them and go back to the house through the garden. On the way back you are hit on the head by a leaf. It falls to the ground where you see it as a yellow leaf. Pick it up and hold it in your left hand.

BO3X ▸ Put your right hand over the left and feel the life in the leaf. Remove the right hand and see the leaf partially green; replace the right hand and feel the life in the leaf, then remove your right hand and see the leaf more green; replace the right hand over the leaf again and feel the life in the leaf, then remove your right hand and see the leaf fully green. Now take the newly born green leaf and put it on your heart. Feel the sap surging through the leaf into the heart, rejuvenating it and sense the new life pulsing through the heart and into the muscles and arteries. Feel and sense the drops of sap descending into the deep life-giving centers of the body, giving youth and vibrating everywhere.

Note: This Green Leaf exercise can be used for healing any ailment. In place of the heart, imagine taking the bright green leaf and putting it on any ailment, stating its place in or on your body. Then feel the leaf's sap running through it. Continue the exercise to the end.

....

THE JOYFUL HEART

BO3X ▸ See, sense, and feel your heart light as a feather.

BO1X ▸ See, sense, and feel your heart singing like a flute.

BO1X ▸ See, sense, and feel your heart flying like the wings of an angel.

BO3X ▸ Into the mirror, see all the images in the above exercises that have touched you. See your attitudes in front of these images and correct them, if necessary.

Personal Renewal:
For Physical Healing

"In a fragrant garden I met one night when my heart was Clear,
What I recognize as Spirit of Delight...He takes my hand.
We have walked all the night...in the fragrant garden...
But in me is always alive the Smiling Spirit of Delight."
-Colette, "In a Fragrant Garden"

ENTERING THE GARDEN

BO3X ► Imagine the blocks in your organs.

BO1X ► Imagine how you have brought the blocks hiding inside you and feel them like a heavy armor.

BO1X ► Imagine how you are walking with this heavy burden along a wall. Behind it is a garden. You reach the closed gate of the garden and try to look at the garden.

BO3X ► See how you stand still in front of the gate and you undo the armor piece by piece, saying in your mind loudly the name of one of your difficulties or disorders and throwing each piece of the armor behind you.

BO1X ► Open the gate, if it has not opened by itself.

BO1X ► Enter the garden. When walking in the garden, find the fountain. Bend down to it or stretch up to it. Wash your hands and your face, and cupping your hands drink of this clear, nourishing, and purifying water.

BO1X ► Look at yourself. How is your hair? How are you dressed? How do you feel?

BO3X ► See yourself climbing up a branch of the Tree of Life. What do you see, feel, and know when returning to The Origin?

BO1X ► Being always on the Tree of Life, see Abraham receiving the three angels.

BO3X ► Sense the parts of your body that are weaker, congested, depleted. Look for the hot, cold, irregular tingling from electrical charges. Allow your hands to massage the areas of tension, making full contact. Be totally aware of the area of your body where your hands are feeling areas of tension.

RENEWAL

BO3X ▸ See and sense by means of the physical body how you are working at your best on a sport you like.

BO1X ▸ See how this form of concentration on the body is involving all your being.

BO1X ▸ Sense in your body all the movements you are doing. Recognize the signal that you sense, see, and hear when doing well.

BO1X ▸ See and know how winning is performing well with others.

BO1X ▸ See and feel in your body how you have your emotional center controlled.

BO3X ▸ See and know where in your body has been an error. Setting aside your thoughts, know in your body the new sensations when performing again after the error has been made clear.

BO3X ▸ Stand between two mirrors, a clear one before you; a circular, convex, black mirror behind you. Looking into the clear mirror, see your whole body. Now turn your head 180 degrees and look downward at the reflection of your back in the black mirror.

BO1X ▸ See where in your body anger resides.

BO1X ▸ Clean out the black mirror from right to left with the circular motion of the forefinger of your left hand, eradicating shame, guilt, fear, and regret. Now turn your head 180 degrees, facing forward. Looking into the clear mirror, see where love resides in your body. Where does joy reside?

BO3X ▸ Where in your body does your father reside? Take him out respectfully. Where in your body does your mother reside? Remove her sweetly. What do you sense after each removal?

BO3X ▸ Find other areas in your body holding some emotional charge or block. What messages are these giving?

BO3X ▸ Draw a map on your body, showing areas of blockage. What message does your body give to you? Note the possible difficulty when doing this exercise. What may those areas say if they could speak? How do you respond? What message is being sent to you by each area? What do they ask for?

OPENING THE CLOSED SPHINCTER DOORS

BO3X ▸ Sense and feel together the anal, genital, mouth, and eye muscles opening and contracting the circular fibers. REPEAT PHYSICALLY

BO3X ▸ Sense how your throat is playing you the messages from the other centers and hear your voice as the messenger with yourself and others. REPEAT PHYSICALLY

BO3X –Sense how your throat is bringing all the messages of yourself and others.

BO3X ▸ See how when closing the mouth, you change your structure and are unable to speak and to learn by heart.

BO1X ▸ Sense that your memory is stopped.

BO1X ▸ See how as a child our emotions are different. We are more angry and loving than others.

BO1X ▸ See and know how language and emotions are used to choreograph a beautiful ballet by sounds and gestures.

BO3X ▸ As a baby, see how sensations as words to you such as "good child, eat, smile" are associated with warm touch.

MYOMERES
(MUSCULAR RINGS AROUND THE BODY)

BO3X ▸ See the rings of the body corresponding to groups of vertebrae. See and sense one ring at the level of the lumbar spine. See and sense the cervical vertebrae at the level of the neck from the first to the seventh vertebrae.

BO1X ▸ See, know, and discover what is happening in your body. See and feel what is the segment that is more sensitive. See and find what is the calmer segment. See and feel what is the quieter one.

BOX1 ▸ See and recognize clearly what is the color of your cervical vertebrae. See and recognize clearly the colors of your lumbar vertebrae.

JOURNEY INTO THE SELF

BO3X ▸ Explore and discover the iceberg hidden under the surface. In this journey be conscious of how your body is responding in areas far from the area you are touching.

BO1X ▸ Now with your two forefingers, simultaneously touch both these places, the one you have touched directly and the one reacting in response. Touch sweetly these two places to imprint the sensations. Sense the spots or areas of concentrated pain, discomfort, and pleasure. Now press only the reactive part. See, feel, and sense what happens.

RELIEF OF TENSION AND SYMPTOMS

BO3X ▸ VISUAL: Contract the ocular muscles. Then exert pressure on the eyes.

BO1X ▸ REPEAT PHYSICALLY.

BO3X ▸ ORAL: Iron the muscles of the neck and flatten them. Feel 1,000 muscles involved in speech.

BO3X ▸ CERVICAL: Turn the cervical vertebrae 180 degrees, one at a time, going from the seventh to the Atlas 180 degrees and going back again, one at a time.

BO3X ▸ DIAPHRAGM: Loosen the diaphragm by any means you wish.

BO3X ▸ ABDOMINALS: Open the abdomen.

BO3X ▸ PELVIC: Loosen and cleanse all the pelvic bones and cavity.

TURNING THE BONES
TO MAKE THEM REMEMBER

BO1X ▸ Starting from the coccyx, see each vertebra turn 180 degrees and become glistening white and turn back again full of light.

BO3X ▸ See the hip bones rotate, become glistening white and filled with light.

BO1X ▸ Starting from the feet, see all the leg bones turning, become glistening white and filled with light.

BO1X ▸ See the bones of the arms and hands rotating, become glistening white and turning back filled with light.

BO1X ▸ See the shoulder bones turn, become glistening white and turn back filled with light.

BO3X ▸ See your spine of light move out of your body and dance gently and then seeing the sternum filled with light and dancing with the spinal column.

EYES OF THE HEART:
QUEST OF PEOPLE WITH VISION

BO3X ▸ Sense your heart.

BO1X ▸ Feel the marvel of how it is palpitating and dilating.

BO1X ▸ See and sense your heart enlightened and shining as a star.

BO1X ▸ See the eye of your heart with its radiating light. Let this clear light guide you into deep night.

BO1X ▸ Imagine your ear as an eye.

BO1X ▸ See with this ear how and what you see.

BO1X ▸ Now your eyes are becoming ears. Listen to what your eyes are hearing. Pay attention to the direction of the sound.

BO3X ▸ See with your eyes, ears, hands, and feet.

BO1X ▸ See with the eyes of your eyes, ears, hands, and feet and hear with your body, seeing all over.

BO3X ▸ Imagine the world divided into the smallest segments. They are all segmented and whole at the same time. Know and see the eyes of the bodies, each seeing whole.

BO1X ▸ Find a seat for yourself in a night as clear as a day. Sense the density of darkness. Find and see it as if it is noon. See that in this day/night, the night cannot decline.

- -

SORTIE OF THE BODY

BO3X ▸ From the top of your house look at your body descending the back staircase. Know how all you choose to be is contained in your own form. See yourself complete and perfect.

BO1X ▸ Climbing up the front stairs of the house to the bedroom, see yourself going to bed, sleeping quietly in your perfect form.

BO1X ▸ Lying in your bed, see yourself extending your arms and sensing objects that are farther than you habitually reach. See yourself extending your arms and hands to reach and sense farther and farther objects in the room, the house, outside the house. Try to recognize each object by your sensations.

BO1X ▸ Return your arms to your bed by the same way.

- -

BODY PREPARATION

BO3X ▸ See yourself as a rhythmic one going from source to source. See how all the parts of the body-reality are a version in flesh of the soul's reality.

BO1X ▸ Sense how all the segments of your internal universe are reflected within the outer universe.

BO1X ▸ Sense and know that to study the human soul and to learn how to know it, you have to study your body's inside anatomy.

BO1X ▸ Sense and feel peace as a tranquil soul submission.

BO1X ▸ Sense and feel how the study of your body is a key to the nature of God and the universe.

TO MAINTAIN EQUILIBRIUM

BO3X ▸ See and know how to recognize what bodes danger. Know how to banish it by means of timely precautions.

BO1X ▸ See and know how a strong man or woman does not allow themselves to be infected by the general intoxications.

BO1X ▸ See and sense yourself checking this course.

BO3X ▸ See and know what it means not to throw yourself away in the world.

BO3X ▸ See and know how by tranquilly waiting, you develop your personal worth by your own efforts.

BO1X ▸ Know how what is yours cannot be permanently lost.

BO1X ▸ See and sense yourself being careful all day long.

BO1X ▸ See, sense, and know how by being careful and thoughtful you may avert evil consequences.

EXISTING IS RESISTING: MOSES

BO3X ▸ See and feel the truth of what is told to Moses as a newborn by the midwife, "You are now responsible for your life as I am responsible for mine."

BO3X ▸ See, feel, and recognize how spilling honey onto a painful spot of emotion is quieting and increasing the general energy.

BO3X ▸ Hear and tell to yourself what is told to the one becoming an adult. "Now that you are an elder, drop your weapons and instead use your mind and wisdom."

BO3X ► Live and feel in yourself the meaning of Moses saying, "What we on earth as society accept, God above will have no choice but to accept."

EXISTING IS RESISTING:
FROM GRAND RAPIDS INDIANS

BO3X ► See and know how you, as a perfect human being in the image of God, have the right, duty, and knowledge to perfect each day the work performed by wind and water.

BO3X ► See and recognize how you have already seen that aging is only a struggle that has to be fought.

BO3X ► See yourself fighting against the dancing tiger until it is changed into a cat.

FOR CHILDREN SUFFERING PAIN
(TO BE DONE BY THE CHILD)

BO3X ► See into the red place of a pain. Call after the jaguar ogre. See it running to you and swallowing the red pain. Thank him and ask him to return quickly and nicely when there is another pain.

CHRONIC ILLNESS IN CHILDREN
(TO BE DONE FOR THE CHILD)

BO3X ▶ See the struggle of the Children of Darkness and the Children of Light.

BO1X ▶ See, feel, and live how the Children of Light are pushing away the Children of Darkness.

MINDBODY HEALING

BO3X ▶ See and feel some of your inappropriate or incorrect reactions of mindbody emotions.

BO1X ▶ See, feel, and know how they may be repaired.

BO1X ▶ See how they may become an integrated response to the reality of others.

BO3X ▶ See and live what is uniting the world together.

BO3X ▶ Look at the premises that are written in the seven days of creation in Genesis. See yourself looking at it from a star.

BO3X ▶ See and feel how it is connected with the former premises.

BO3X ▶ See and feel how you are curing yourself with each First Becoming. Feel and know in yourself of the creative activity of each First Becoming.

BO3X ▶ See, sense, and recognize in yourself the Becoming of Life. Know how it is all-powerful.

BO1X ▶ Live this premise totally.

Body Work

"From multiplicity this is bringing Oneness. Being united, we become one and our mind is the One Mind."
-Colette, "The Only Mind"

SPORT AND DANCE: UNITING BODY AND SOUL

BO3X ▸ See how by physical bodywork or the sport you like, you are performing at the best of all your possibilities.

BO3X ▸ See how this form of concentration on your body is involving all your being.

BO3X ▸ Sense in your body all the movements you are doing. Recognize the signal you do or hear when doing well.

BO3X ▸ Having well performed, see that another is winning. See and feel in all your body how or whether you have your emotions under control.

BO3X ▸ See and know where the error has been and how by opening your mind you are performing at the top of yourself. Feel in your body the new sensations when performing with joy after an error has been cleared.

BO3X ▸ See and know how your perfected body is now a fit habitation for your soul.

BO3X ▸ See and feel how someone is cleansing your soul.

BO3X ▸ See and feel how you are cleansing your soul and feel how you are expelling fears.

BO1X ▸ See and feel how you are cleansing your soul and feel how you are discarding worn out desires.

BO1X ▸ See and feel how you are cleansing your soul and live how you are forgetting frustration.

BO1X ▸ See and feel how you are cleansing your soul and sense your resentment peeled away.

The Body Out of Your Body

"...Then, feeling in your soul,
a spark of the World Soul—
Only when this is done, your eyes,
are becoming the windows of your soul."
-Colette, "Divination"

THE PEACH OF PERFECTION

BO3X ▸ See yourself standing under a peach tree picking a peach and feeling it in your hands, its texture, scent, and overall weight. Have the peach in your two hands to the width of your shoulders, seeing if there are any spots or blemishes. Clean them with your fingers. See the skin becoming transparent. Allow the peach to return to its size. Put the peach back on the tree.

BO3X ▸ Standing beneath the peach tree, pick a peach. Have it expanding with you and sense what is your most comfortable position. Return the peach to its size. Put it back on the tree.

BO3X ▸ Pick a peach. See the core and the flesh around the core growing and expanding beyond the possible. Look at yourself from the outside.

BO3X ▸ In your room there is a peach on your desk. Watch it growing. Become one with it. Walk around the table, a little above it. Watch it from all directions. Find the most comfortable distance.

BO4X ▸ See yourself in your mother's womb sucking your thumb swimming in the waters.

BO4X ▸ You are in your mother's womb. Your mouth is not formed for eating. You are eating through your umbilical cord. Know what the mouth is for.

OSIRIS/ISIS ▸ EXISTING AND RESISTING: TO RE-PAIR THE BODY

BO3X ▸ See and know the world as it is at this point. Now see how Osiris, the God of Death and the God of Spring, Growth, and Resurrection have been in conflict.

BO1X ▸ See how Isis repairs Osiris and makes him renewed by putting him in the trunk of a tree to live the life of the tree.

BO3X ▸ See and know what sort of genesis is coming from chaos.

BO3X ▸ See and live how doing things too quickly makes you sick.

BO1X ▸ Hear and see how when out of time, the right repair is to learn how to play and sing in time.

BO3X ▸ See and live in yourself as a story or a tale, the nine lives of a cat. Find the key for survival in renewing yourself.

BO3X ▸ Feel how a wonder tale is making you more alive.

BO3X ▸ See yourself as a prehistoric hunter, hunting with the sun behind him and his shadow in front of him. Know how when you and your shadow have joined, you are successful and whole.

BO3X ▸ See a big, high fire sometimes referred to as St. Elmo's Fire*. See yourself jumping over the fire. What do you feel?

BO3X ▸ See, sense, feel, and know that you do not find God in the storm but in the quietness.

BO3X ▸ See pain as a favor, a boon.

BO1X ▸ See and feel it as the means by which our inner system is guiding us to well-being.

Exercises in Renewal

"Once more, has appeared this "Perfect Nature"
Coming with Triumph and Glory…"
-Colette, "The Being of Light"

DESTINY

BO3X ▸ In a garden find a spade. Use it to find something you need.

BO3X ▸ See an animal.

BO1X ▸ See two upset animals. What happens?

BO1X ▸ See an animal coming toward you on an incline.

BO3X ▸ Herd wild horses into a corral.

BO1X ▸ Defuse a live bomb.

BO1X ▸ Go backwards through a wallpapered wall.

BO3X ▸ You are at the entrance of the birth canal, head pressed downward. What is happening?

BO3X ▸ Into a mirror see what you would most dislike to know or hear about yourself. Correct it.

BO1X ▸ Into a mirror write your name. See what it is becoming or turning into.

BO1X ▸ Listen to the sound your name makes.

BO3X ▸ You are wrapped in bandages up to your neck. How do you feel? Unwrap them and make a ball. What happens?

REJUVENATION

BO3X ► Go backwards into a panther or a leopard skin. What happens?

BO3X ► There are three doors, a left, a middle, and a right.

BO1X ► Go through the left door. What do you discover?

BO1X ► Go through the middle door. What do you discover?

BO1X ► Go through the right door. What do you discover?

FOR CATCHING TIME

BO3X ► Say to whom your love feelings belong.

BO1X ► Say to whom your time belongs.

BO1X ► Say to whom your life belongs.

LABYRINTH: COMING TO THE CENTER OF SELF

BO3X ► You are at the entrance to a labyrinth. Have with you a ball of red or golden thread to lay along the center to find your way out. Going to the center, discover what you find there for yourself. Return by the way you have come. Note the different feelings going and returning.

EVOLUTION

BO3X ► See two insects. What do you feel? See two fish. What do you feel? See two amphibians. What do you feel?

BO1X ▶ See two reptiles. What do you feel? See two birds. What do you feel? See two mammals. What do you feel? See two humans. What do you feel?

WHAT YOU HAVE NOT LIVED SUFFICIENTLY AND NEEDS TO BE LIVED NOW: TO CLEAR UP THE PAST

BO1X ▶ Be in a classroom. Live your experience there in a new way.

BO1X ▶ Be in a playground. Live your experience there in a new way.

BO3X ▶ Hold an object in each hand. Then change the object to the opposite hand. What happens?

BO1X ▶ See someone of your own sex in front of you. What do you feel?

BO1X ▶ See someone of the opposite sex in front of you. What do you feel?

BO3X ▶ Sacrifice a part of yourself. What happens?

TO FIND THE HIGHER, ESSENTIAL ASPECTS OF YOURSELF

BO3X ▶ Wind a golden thread into a ball. Absorb yourself into it.

BO3X ▶ See yourself as a seed becoming a tree and then reverse into a seed.

BO1X ▶ A wheel is spinning in the abdomen.

BO1X ▸ See and feel the essence of Buddhism.

BO1X ▸ See yourself turning the wheel.

BO3X ▸ See two spirals standing point to point. What is your experience?

....

UNITING EXERCISES

Preparation:

BO3X ▸ See yourself in a mirror that has handles.

BO1X ▸ Hear a conch shell and a lyre and listen to the sounds.

BO1X ▸ See a vase filled with flowers.

BO1X ▸ See a cup filled with cookies.

BO1X ▸ There's a silk object before you. Touch it.

BO1X ▸ Smell a jar of mixed spices.

Then...

BO1X ▸ Unite cold and heat.

BO1X ▸ Unite left and right.

BO1X ▸ Unite dry and wet.

BO1X ▸ Unite rest and activity.

BO1X ▸ Unite passing and permanent.

BO1X ▸ Unite in and out.

BO1X ▸ Unite earth and air.

BO1X ▸ Unite fast and slow.

BO1X ▸ Unite physical and spiritual.

BO7X ▸ COUNTING BACKWARDS FROM 7 TO 1 WITH AN OUT-BREATH ON EACH NUMBER. At 1, see exactly how to control exaggeration.

BO1X ▸ See yourself in front of an audience exaggerating and bursting forth. Looking into a mirror, see if you like your face or the face you see. If not, see the face you want.

REMOVING NEGATIVE OR DISTRESSING FEELINGS

BO3X ► Spit into a glass of water. Afterwards, swallow the water.

BO3X ► Have your double there. Hug and kiss it.

BO3X ► Be on the back porch of a house. Have a broom and sweep out all the debris from the porch. Sweep it into a pile adjacent to the porch. When you finish sweeping the pile into a trash bag, take the bag to the far end of the lawn. Digging a hole near a large rock, put the bag on the rock and burn it. Bury the ashes in the hole. Come back to the porch. See it again. How do you feel?

....

INTO THE MIRRORS:
TO SEE LACKS AND LIMITATIONS

BO3X ► Into the mirror see your lacks and limitations. Correct them. If you are not able, push them out of the mirror to the left.

BO1X ► See guilts and rejections. Correct them. If you are not able, push them out of the mirror to the left.

BO1X ► See envy and acquisitiveness. Correct them. If you are not able, push them out of the mirror to the left.

BO1X ► See insecurity and uncertainty. Correct them. If you are not able, push them out of the mirror to the left.

BO1X ► See repression and frustration. Correct them. If you are not able, push them out of the mirror to the left.

BO1X ► See hostility and resentment. Correct them. If you are not able, push them out of the mirror to the left.

BO1X ► See greed and futility. Correct them. If you are not able, push them out of the mirror to the left.

BO1X ► See fear and timidity. Correct them. If you are not able, push them out of the mirror to the left.

BO1X ► See hatred and anger. Correct them. If you are not able, push them out of the mirror to the left.

BO1X ▸ See and get rid of pain and self-affliction. If you are not able, push them out of the mirror to the left.

BO1X ▸ See yourself in front of sadness and despair. Correct them. If you are not able to make a correction, push them out of the mirror to the left.

ABRAHAM: BREAKING THE IDOLS

BO3X ▸ Live the breaking of idols as Abraham did.

BO3X ▸ Feel and know in yourself the total change and the newness when breaking with the commonly accepted way of life.

BO3X ▸ Hear and see Abraham telling God, "Hineni" (Hee Nay Nee), [from the Hebrew], "Here I am" or "I am Coming."

BO3X ▸ Hear and feel the reverberation of the sound "Hee Nay Nee."

BO3X ▸ Live and know how the sound "Hee Nay Nee" is the key that can open the fifty doors of the palace and is always opening them.

BO3X ▸ Live and know how by crossing the bridge you are crossing the Red Sea, jumping over the abyss or altogether breaking the idols.

BO1X ▸ See and feel how by traveling you are reaching the source of the river. See, sense, feel, and know how you are walking on the wings of the wind.

BO1X ▸ Know and sense how all that was potential is now reality and is already present with you, always in you.

BO1X ▸ See and choose your own way. Have a blueprint of it and go ahead.

BO1X ▸ Sense how all in your life is welcomed and how you are teaching Isaac to laugh because life is simple and you are smiling at it.

JONAH: ESCAPING DESTINY

BO3X ▸ Imagine being on a boat escaping from your destiny. A storm arises and assaults the boat. Go overboard into a whale. Spend three days there healing. The whale is whisking you through the water and throwing you onto dry land.

BO1X ▸ On land, sit under a tree and accept to take on your direction, seeing yourself healthy and whole.

BO1X ▸ Know what sacrifice has to be made for the direction and accept it.

Coming Into Order

"Going out of myself we meet
On a high ladder made of crowns of letters."
-Colette, "Crowns of Letters"

GUILT AND REPENTANCE*:
FROM RABBI ADIN STEINSALTZ*

BO3X ► See and live how repentance is not contrition or regret for error or fault.

BO1X ► Know why the sages have included repentance among the entities created before the world itself was created.

BO3X ► Live repentance as a universal primordial phenomenon.

BO1X ► See it as the restructuring of the world.

BO1X ► Know how before human beings were created, we were given the possibility of changing the course of our life by choosing freely.

BO1X ► Live and know how by repentance you are extricating yourself from the web and chain of causality that is for you the path of no return.

BO1X ► Live and know how by repentance you have a possibility of control over your existence including time.

BO3X ► Live and know how even in cases when the past is fixed, you have the possibility of changing its means and by repentance there is the potential for something else.

BO3X ► Feel and sense how we may feel guilt only if we refuse to assume a part of the burden of the world.

BO3X ► See and know how if God has felt very good when creating humans and has said that humans are very good, we cannot be guilty to be a human being with all of our duties, obligations, and servitudes.

BO3X ► Know in yourself that you cannot feel guilty for your personal errors, faults, and mistakes, if you are trying to repair them at all levels: mental, moral, emotional.

BO3X ► Feel and know how repentance is a process that can affect real change in the world by severing the effects of one's transgressions.

BO1X ► Sense and know how repentance is an attempt to nullify or alter the past, shattering the order of our own existence.

BO1X ► Sense and know how repentance is breaking through the ordinary limits of the self and becoming ever renewed by extricating from causality.

BO1X ► Know how it is the absence of the sense of guilt or despair that is permitting you to leap over the past.

BO3X ► Know how you have the power to break your uncompromising fate by changing your past, your goals, and aims.

BO3X ► See and know how injuries or sins are existing as such only in time, even with a changed or altered past and present.

BO1X ► See that the earlier acts and their consequences are not obliterated.

BO1X ► Feel and see how it is by the repair or reparation that the significance of the past is changed. See how by doing so, you reach a higher level.

BO1X ► See and know how the first stage of reparation is to complete and balance the picture of your life.

BO3X ► Return quickly backwards into life from now to five years old by completing and repairing what needs to be repaired and perfectly cleaning what stays after the repair.

BO1X ► Sense and see how you have to build and create yourself anew by changing the order of good and evil.

BO1X ► Feel and see how the totality of your life is receiving then an instruction of positive value.

BO3X ► Feel and know how you create the possibility for your creations and transgressions to be your merits.

BO3X ► See, feel, and know that you have the possibility to fall again and again and then to transform more and more segments of your life.

BO3X ► Feel and sense how your guilt at falling increases your will and power to do good instead of reducing your status and sapping your strength. Know how you are reversing yourself and from separation you are returning to unity.

BO1X ► Live how false guilt often is inverted pride coming from weakness, which is as much physical as it is emotional.

BO1X ► Sense and know how by going out of false guilt and false humility you are entering a different form of pain that is no longer a weight, but is the piercing sword.

BO1X ► Sense and feel how you return to real innocence by accepting some sacrifice and self-recognition.

BO3X ► Sense, feel, and see how going out of false guilt, remorse, and blame, the loss of vital energy is returned to you.

BO1X ► Sense and know how true guilt feelings are always an evasion of objective awareness in taking on personal responsibility.

BO3X ► Live the sufferings of the innocent Job that are bringing you nearer to God by healing the split between curse and blessing.

GUILTY OF INNOCENCE

BO3X ► Confess to your heart five errors you are feeling guilty of.

BO1X ► See, sense, and feel that God forgives you and that you forgive yourself completely.

BO3X ► Find your grief. Tie it up in your heart.

SHADOW BEINGS

BO3X ► Know that God created the shadow beings on the twilight of the sixth day. They are remaking outside bodies in the shadowy matter.

BO1X ► See yourself blowing at them very strongly, telling them to go away.

BO3X ► Experience the shadow beings inside you. See your stomach secreting the acid juice that dissolves them. Sense them being destroyed in the small intestine and expel them into the toilet. Flush three times. Then take a shower. What do you sense and feel?

THE CASTLE

BO3X ► See yourself dressed in white armor and riding a white horse.

BO1X ▸ Know your mission is to conquer a castle single-handedly. When you succeed, then.

BO1X ▸ Know that all castles have a special room. Find the special room and see who or what is in the room and what happens.

BO1X ▸ Now that you have found your special room, go to the dungeon and see what is there. Hear the message this being has to tell you. Free it and send it on its way.

BO1X ▸ After freeing the being, know that every Lord of the Castle keeps a Book of Reason where he would keep daily notes of what was important for posterity. See the book and read what is written for yesterday. Then inscribe something for today. After that, see the inscription that will be there tomorrow.

BO1X ▸ See yourself on your white horse wearing your white armor on your way to new adventures.

CLEANSING THE BRAIN: TO REMOVE OLD EMOTIONS, GUILT AND RESENTMENT

BO3X ▸ Wash your hair with shampoo and lots of sparkling water. If any section is not bright enough, see how the light from above makes it shine. Now clean the inside of your head by cutting the cranium delicately as if it were a box. Remove the top and put your hair inside, with the hair sweeping away all the old emotions, guilt, and feelings of resentment. When it is clean, put the top back on and glue it carefully. Then wash the hair once again.

REMOVING THE FOREIGN PRESENCE

BO3X ▸ Look at yourself in a mirror saying, "To whom have I a pain, burden, or disturbance?" Into the mirror, touch each part of your body beginning with the neck and shoulders asking, "Who is disturbing this part of me? Who is irritating me?" Touch the body all the way down in the mirror and see the hidden one appear. See whom you are to forgive and ask to be forgiven.

THE SWORD: FOR RESENTMENT

BO1X ▸ Feel resentment like a sword going through you and piercing the one you resent. Sense and feel what appears.

BALANCING FEELINGS

BO1X ▸ Sense in front of you a person you love, one to whom you feel indifferent and one you resent. Have them change places until you can balance your feelings and fulfill the commandment of Loving Your Neighbor As Yourself.

KNIGHT OF ARMOR:
FOR TAKING CHARGE OF GUILT

BO3X ▸ Imagine you are carrying all the weight of your guilt and resentment on you like a metallic armor. Nothing can rid you of it. Someone tells you that if you can get access into the Garden of Eden, there is a little lake where at the junction of four rivers the water is so clean it cleanses everything.

BO1X ▸ In spite of your heavy armor, you are walking toward the Garden of Eden. Leave the city and go into a valley. On one side you have a cliff. On the other you can see the ocean at a distance.

BO1X ▸ You are now walking on a very narrow path bordered by a wall. Over the path you can see beautiful trees of different scents. A very pleasant fragrance is streaming from the trees.

BO1X ▸ You now arrive at the entrance of the Garden. You are facing a very long gate. You try opening the gate but cannot. You are now tired because the weight of your heavy armor is exhausting. You begin to have difficulty breathing so you remove the helmet and throw it behind you. Then you remove the armor from your body and arms and throw them over your shoulders. Now that your arms are free, you feel better, and you want to free your legs. You begin by freeing the knees. And after that you remove the pieces covering your calves and thighs, throwing all of the parts over your shoulders. When you remove your boots you are completely light and agile. You then go to the gate. Your hand is ready to open it, when the gate opens on its own. Go through and say thank you. If it does not open, open it and describe what you see.

BO1X ▸ You are now walking on a very smooth path. You find the lake. Describe it.

BO1X ▸ Dive into the water three times, each time staying under the water as long as you can hold your breath. The third time, look at the bottom of the water to find something that is there for you.

BO1X ▸ And leave the water. What are you wearing? How does your body look? What have you found? Now choose a tree that appeals to you and sit underneath it. Look at the living beings around you, the insects and the birds.

BO1X ▸ And look at what you have brought up from the depths of the water. You become whole again and feel yourself at a higher level beyond the level of time and space.

BO1X ▸ And take a walk around the garden. Look at the flowers and fill yourself with the beauty of the garden. Now leave the garden and go to rest at the edge of the sea. Sit there and rest while you watch the pleasure of the children on the beach. Look at the beauty of the ocean and the infinity of the sky.

....

ONE HEART

BO3X ▸ See yourself at Mount Sinai wanting with all your heart to hear God. You know for that you need to reach the level of total unity with every other person present. All must be like one person with one heart.

BO1X ▸ If you are unable to feel this unity, there is resentment of the one you resist, who is next to you. You will be physically there, but not feel the ecstatic joy of the love union. Rise to that feeling of unity and feel the life-giving force flooding you.

GLOSSARY OF TERMS

James Allen (1864-1912) ▸ British author who believed in the power of thought to change one's beliefs and actions. "A man is literally what he thinks, his character being the complete sum of all his thoughts."

Angst ▸ German word for fear/anxiety used in English to describe an intense feeling of strife. Derived from the Latin angustia, meaning "tensity, tightness," and angor, meaning "chocking, clogging". Angst differs from fear in that it refers to non-directional emotion rather than material threat and reflects a feeling of fear towards anything strange or unfamiliar.

Archangel Raphael ▸ Archangel of Healing in Judaism, Christianity, and Islam.

Bachya ben Joseph ibn Pakuda ▸ 11th century Spanish Jewish philosopher, jurist, and mystic. Bahya considered it more important for a man to love God in his heart than to seek to know God through his intellect and opposed an anthropomorphic conception of God.

Bodhidharma ▸ Early 5th century Buddhist monk, originally from Southern India, traditionally credited as the transmitter of Zen to China.

Thorlief Boman ▸ Norwegian biblical scholar who explained that the Israelites, unlike Europeans or people in the West, did not understand time as something measurable.

The Cloud of Unknowing ▸ Late 14th century, anonymous Christian mystical text. A spiritual guide to contemplative prayer and the esoteric techniques and meanings of late medieval monasticism. The book counsels a young student not to seek God through knowledge but through what the author speaks of as a "naked intent" and a "blind love."

Alexandra David-Neel (1868-1969) ▸ Belgian-French explorer, anarchist, spiritualist, Buddhist, and writer famous for her visit to Lhasa, Tibet, in 1924, which was closed to foreigners at the time.

Pierre Teilhard de Chardin (1881-1955) ▸ 20th Century French, Jesuit priest, spiritual sage and scientist.

Djinni (Genie) ▸ In Islam and pre-Islamic Arabian folklore, a supernatural creature, either good or evil, possessing free will. Currently refers to a magical spirit often evoked by gestures, such as rubbing a bottle or lamp, who performs at the master's bidding.

Larry Dossey (b. 1940) ▸ Texas physician, deeply rooted in the scientific world, who has become an internationally influential advocate of the role of the mind in health and the role of spirituality in healthcare.

Durga (Maa Durga or Mother Durga) ▸ Hindu goddess ("the inaccessible" or "the invincible") who is a form of Devi, the supremely radiant goddess She is depicted as having ten arms, riding a lion or a tiger, carrying weapons (including a Lotus flower), maintaining a meditative smile, and practicing mudras, or symbolic hand gestures. An embodiment of creative feminine force (Shakti), she exists in a state of svätantrya (dependence on the universe and nothing/nobody else, i.e., self-sufficiency) and fierce compassion. Durga is considered by Hindus to be an aspect of Kali, thus considered the fiercer, demon-fighting form of Shiva's wife, goddess Parvati. She manifests fearlessness and patience, and never loses her sense of humor, even during spiritual battles of epic proportion.

Egyptian Ka ▸ One of five parts of the human soul, the Ka is the life force or that which distinguishes the difference between a living and dead person, with death occurring when it leaves the body. The Ka was often represented in Egyptian iconography as a second image of the individual, e.g. a double. Egyptians believed that certain gods created each person's Ka, breathing it into them at the instant of their birth, similar to the concept of spirit. Believing that the Ka was sustained through food and drink, the Egyptians presented food and drink to the dead.

Elijah (E-li-Ja-hu – "My God is Yahweh") ▸ 9th Century BCE prophet in Israel, whose name appears in the Old and New Testaments and the Qur'an. According to the *Book of Kings,* he raised the dead, brought fire down from the sky, and ascended to heaven in a chariot. *The Book of Malachi* (3:23) prophesied Elijah's return as harbinger of the Messiah.

Isis ▸ Egyptian goddess of wisdom, motherhood, fertility and simplicity, from whom all beginnings arose. Sister and wife of Osiris and mother of Horus, she was the first daughter of Geb, god of the Earth, and Nut, the goddess of the Overarching Sky. Isis was instrumental in the resurrection of Osiris when she used her magical skills to restore the murdered Osiris' body to life after she gathered the body parts that had been strewn about the earth by his murderer Seth. In later myths, ancient Egyptians believed that the Nile River flooded every year because of her tears of sorrow for Osiris. They reenacted the occurrence of his death and rebirth each year through rituals.

Janus ▸ The two-faced Roman god, with one face looking toward the future, the other to the past. It is often represented by one face (past) looking depressed and pessimistic, the other (future) looking cheerful and optimistic.

Kabir ▸ 14th century Indian saint and mystic, composer and poet, whose literature has greatly influenced the Indian Bhakti movement. According to Kabir, all life is an interplay of two spiritual principles – the personal soul (Jivatma) and God (Paramatma). Salvation is the process of bringing these two divine principles into union. His straightforward philosophies often advocated leaving aside Islamic and Hindu religious texts to follow the Simple/Natural Way to oneness in God. His greatest poetic work is the Bijak (the "Seedling"), an idea of the fundamental One.

Sam Keen (b. 1931) ▸ American author and philosopher whose best-known work is *Fire in the Belly: On Being a Man.*

Count Herman Keyserling (1880-1946) ▸ The first Western thinker to conceive of and promote a planetary culture, beyond nationalism and cultural ethnocentrism, based on recognition of the equal value and validity of non-western cultures and philosophies. He is the author of many books including *The Travel Diary of a Philosopher.*

Kumbh Mela ▸ A mass Hindu pilgrimage which occurs every three years, rotating across the following four locations: the confluence of the Ganges, Yamuna, and mythical Saraswati Rivers; at Haridwar along the Ganges River; at Ujjain along the Kshipra River; and at Nashik along the Godavari River.

R. D. Laing (1927-1989) ▸ British psychiatrist who developed innovative strategies in the treatment of schizophrenia.

Maggid (lit. "narrator") ▸ Hebrew term denoting "one who brings a message" (II Samuel 15:13). To the kabbalists, a maggid was a mysterious voice or agency that communicated secret knowledge to the privileged through dreams or daytime revelations. Most of these strange experiences might today be ascribed to telepathy, extrasensory perception, and kindred factors. From early times, however, the term maggid was synonymous with preacher, who delivered three-part sermons comprising (1) a biblical verse usually chosen from the weekly Torah reading; (2) an exposition of this verse based on homiletics, allegory, parables, and topical comments; (3) and a final message of encouragement ending with Isaiah 59:20 and the recital of the Mourner's Prayer.

Gabriel Garcia Marquez (b. 1928) ▸ South American journalist and novelist, awarded the Nobel Prize in Literature in 1982.

Rabbi Menachem Mendel Morgensztern of Kotzk, better known as the **Kotzker Rebbe** (1787-1859) ▸ A Hasidic leader well known for his incisive and down-to-earth philosophies, and sharp-witted sayings. He appears to have had little patience for false piety or stupidity. He never published any works but wrote many manuscripts, which he had burned before his death. Several collections of his sayings have been published, most notably *Emes VeEmunah* (Truth and Faith).

Rabbi Nachman of Breslov (1772 -1810) ▸ Founder of the Breslov Hasidic dynasty and great-grandson of the Baal Shem Tov. He invigorated the Hasidic movement by combining the esoteric secrets of Kabbalah with in-depth Torah scholarship. The concept of "self seclusion" is central to his thinking and refers to an unstructured, spontaneous, and individualized form of prayer and meditation practiced to establish a close, personal relationship with God and a clearer understanding of one's personal motives and goals.

Nimir ▸ A Norse god.

Osiris ▸ Egyptian god of the afterlife, brother/husband of Isis and father of Horus. He acted as a merciful judge and as the underworld agency granting all life, including sprouting vegetation and the fertile flooding of the Nile River. The Kings of Egypt (and later all Egyptians) were associated with Osiris in death: as Osiris rose from the dead, they would, in union with him, inherit eternal life through a process of imitative magic. Osiris was viewed as the one who died to save the many and who rose from the dead, the first of a long line of resurrected beings that have influenced man's beliefs in and expectations of eternal life.

Plotinus ▸ 3rd century mystic considered the founder of Neo-Platonism (along with his teacher Ammonius Saccas). The composer of the *Enneads* (edited and compiled by his student Porphyry), whose writings have inspired Pagan, Gnostic, Jewish, Christian, and Islamic metaphysicians and mystics.

Rafuah ▸ Hebrew word for healing.

Wilhelm Reich (1897-1957) ▸ Psychiatrist and psychoanalyst, who focused on character structure rather than neurotic symptoms. Later in life he developed a body psychotherapy that employed touching during sessions as well as the use of the orgone box - a device that accumulated orgone energy, a primordial cosmic energy Reich claimed to have discovered. Today, his work forms the basis of Bio-energetic Analysis, a form of body-oriented psychotherapy that combines psychological analysis, active body work, and relational therapeutic work. The approach includes development of insight/understanding, expression of feelings, and re-establishment of energy flow in the body. A basic tenet of Bioenergetic Analysis is that the body's expressions, posture, patterns of muscular holding, and energetic integrity tell the story of a person's emotional history and shed light on the person's characteristic way of being in the world.

Reliquary ▸ Container for relics (holy items), which may be the physical remains of saints or other religious figures (e.g. bones, pieces of clothing, or some associated object).

Repentance ▸ from the Latin, repentir to feel remorse, contrition or self reproach for what one has done or failed to do. To feel such regret for past conduct as to change one's mind regarding it; to make a change for the better as a result of remorse or contrition for ones errors.

Jules Romains (1885-1972) ▸ French author.

Shu (meaning *dryness* and *he who rises up*) ▸ Egyptian primordial god personifying air, who was created by his father Atum from his breath. With his sister Tefnut (moisture), he fathered Nut, the sky goddess, and Geb (Earth) and held Nut over Geb separating the two. As air, Shu was considered to be a cool, calming influence, a pacifier associated with truth, justice, and order. He is portrayed wearing a headdress with tall feathers and carries an Ankh.

Rabbi Adin Steinsaltz (b. 1937) ▸ Noted rabbi, scholar, philosopher, social critic, and author whose background also includes extensive scientific training. He is known for his popular commentary and translation of both Talmuds into Hebrew, French, Russian, and Spanish. The Rabbi's classic work of Kabbalah, *The Thirteen Petalled Rose,* was first published in 1980. He has authored some

60 books and hundreds of articles on subjects including Talmud, Jewish mysticism, Jewish philosophy, sociology, historical biography, and philosophy.

St. Elmo's Fire ‣ A phenomenon sometimes appearing on ships at sea during thunderstorms. It was regarded by sailors with religious awe for its glowing ball of light, accounting for the name. Physically, St. Elmo's fire is a bright blue or violet glow appearing sometimes from tall, sharply pointed structures such as lightning rods, masts, spires and chimneys, and on aircraft wings. Often accompanying the glow is a distinct hissing or buzzing sound.

Rabindranath Tagore (1861-1941) ‣ Bengali poet, visual artist, playwright, novelist, educationist, social reformer, nationalist, business-manager, and composer who became Asia's first Nobel laureate (1913 ‣ literature). He wrote novels, short stories, songs, dance-dramas, and essays on political and personal topics. Two songs from his canon are now the national anthems of Bangladesh and India.

Third Eye ‣ Pineal gland. Also known as the inner eye. In the Western spiritual tradition the gate leading to the inner realms of higher consciousness. The third eye is often associated with visions, clairvoyance, precognition, and out-of-body experiences.

Third Ventricle *(ventriculus tertius)* ‣ One of four connected cerebrospinal fluid-filled cavities of the ventricular system of the brain.

Three Worlds ‣ The Three Worlds relating to Spirit, Soul and Body.

Transmigration (of the soul) ‣ The idea that after death, the soul, being eternal and immutable, moves into another human form and is reborn, thus imprinting its character on the new body.

Udjat ‣ The Egyptian all-knowing eye of Horus.

White Buffalo Calf Pipe Woman ‣ A sacred woman of supernatural origin, she is treated as a prophet to the extended Lakota Tribe of Teton Sioux American Indians. She brought them a sacred pipe as a reminder of the Creator's Law to live through oneness, love, prayer, good relationship, and to hold all things sacred.

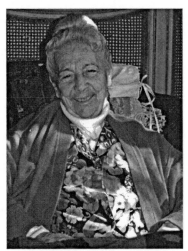

Mme. Colette Aboulker-Muscat

BIOGRAPHIES

Colette Aboulker-Muscat was a psychologist, healer, and spiritual teacher of a unique form of healing called mental imagery. Colette was born into an aristo-cratic Kabbalistic Jewish family in Algeria in the early 1900's. At an early age, her mouth was taped in order to heal a vocal disorder. This forced silence led to her remarkable ability to help others through the power of visualizations. She assisted her father, a prominent surgeon, in treating hopeless cases of wounded soldiers in WW1. She later studied psychology at the Sorbonne. In WWII she and her brother led the North African Resistance against the Nazis. In 1954 she moved to Jerusalem where she devoted her time to healing others by teaching them mental imagery tailored to each sufferer's complaints. She referred to herself as a "teacher of Life" offering visitors her wisdom and insights specific to their individual temperaments and needs.

Her legacy includes *Alone with the One,* a book of poems, and *Mea Culpa: Tales of Resurrection,* a collection of cases of "possession", as well as thousands of her unique and brilliant imagery exercises.

Gerald Epstein, M.D., is one of the foremost practitioners of integrative medicine for healing and transformation. He founded and directs the *American Institute for Mental Imagery* (AIMI), a postgraduate training program for health professionals and an educational center for the public. Dr. Epstein is Assistant Clinical Professor of Psychiatry at Mt. Sinai Medical Center (New York City) and has taught at Colum-bia University's College of Physicians and Surgeons. Initiated into Visionary Kabbal-ah by his teacher Colette Aboulker-Muscat, he is a leading exponent and teacher of the Western spiritual tradition and its application to healing and therapeutics. Dr. Epstein has authored six books and recorded many audios, including the classic reference book *Healing Visualizations: Creating Health Through Imagery* and *The Phoenix Process: One Minute A Day to Health Longevity and Well-Being* (CD). He maintains a private practice in integrative medicine in New York City where he works with individuals, groups and children. To contact Dr. Epstein, call 212-369-4080 or visit: *www.drjerryepstein.org.*

Barbarah L. Fedoroff is a seeker of spiritual truth, a teacher of imagery, and the creator of Inner-Focused Management, a heart-centered approach to work that integrates imagery with sound business practices. Formerly, she served as the CEO of Programs for Parents (PfP), a non-profit organization serving over 8,000 families in New Jersey. In 2009, on the 25th Anniversary of PfP , The New Jersey State Legislature honored her for "her wisdom and expertise."

While with PfP, Barbarah produced and developed the scripts for three video training programs, two winning the Aurora Gold Award "for excellence in the film and video industries": *Identifying Development Delays In Young Children* (2003)*; How Three and Four year Olds Learn in Pre-K* (2006)*;* and the ground-breaking DVD *The Emotional Lives of Infants and Young Children* (2009). She also authored the booklet *Empowering Young Children* that teaches parents and teachers to use imagery with children to deal with the aftermath of 9/11 and other troubling events.

Barbarah is certified in *Imagery, Imagination and Phenomenology* by the *American Institute for Mental Imagery* (AIMI). She is a graduate of The New Seminary, and an ordained Interfaith Minister. Additionally, she is certified in not-for-profit management by Harvard University Business Management for Executives. She offers classes on The *Divine Feminine*, and *Meditations on the Tarot* in Stroudsburg, PA, and posts *Tools for Spiritual Living* that feature audio imagery at: *http://barbarahsblog.wordpress.com/*. Contact her through her website or at *fedzie@ptd.net.*

CPSIA information can be obtained at www.ICGtesting.com
Printed in the USA
LVOW080756060313

322777LV00004B/470/P